T0144192

Spirituality, Health, and Wholeness
An Introductory Guide for Health Care Professionals

THE HAWORTH PRESS
Titles of Related Interest

The Obsessive-Compulsive Disorder: Pastoral Care for the Road to Change by Robert M. Collie

Life Cycle: Psychological and Theological Perceptions by Richard Dayringer

Losses in Later Life: A New Way of Walking with God, Second Edition by R. Scott Sullender

Faith, Spirituality, and Medicine: Toward the Making of the Healing Practitioner by Dana E. King

Aging and Spirituality: Spiritual Dimensions of Aging Theory, Research, Practice, and Policy edited by David O. Moberg

Integrating Spirit and Psyche: Using Women's Narratives in Psychotherapy by Mary Pat Henehan

Mental Health and Spirituality in Later Life edited by Elizabeth MacKinlay

Aging and God: Spiritual Pathways to Mental Health in Midlife and Later Years by Harold G. Koenig

The Power of Spirituality in Therapy: Integrating Spiritual and Religious Beliefs in Mental Health Practice by Peter A. Kahle and John M. Robbins

Bereavement Counseling: Pastoral Care for Complicated Grieving by Junietta Baker McCall

Faith, Medicine, and Science: A Festschrift in Honor of Dr. David B. Larson by Jeff Levin and Harold G. Koenig

Spirituality, Health, and Wholeness
An Introductory Guide for Health Care Professionals

Siroj Sorajjakool, PhD
Henry H. Lamberton, PsyD
Editors

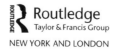

Routledge
Taylor & Francis Group

NEW YORK AND LONDON

First Published by

The Haworth Press, Inc., 10 Alice Street, Binghamton, NY 13904-1580.

Transferred to Digital Printing 2009 by Routledge
270 Madison Ave, New York NY 10016
2 Park Square, Milton Park, Abingdon, Oxon, OX14 4RN

PUBLISHER'S NOTE
Identities and circumstances of individuals discussed in this book have been changed to protect confidentiality.

Chapter 1, "Toward a Theology of Wholeness: A Tentative Model of Whole Person Care" is printed here with permission of The Center for Spiritual Life and Wholeness, Loma Linda University, Loma Linda, CA.

Excerpt from A NIGHT WITHOUT ARMOR: POEMS by JEWEL KILCHER. Copyright© 1998 by Jewel Kilcher. Reprinted by permission of HarperCollins Publishers Inc.

Cover design by Jennifer M. Gaska.

Library of Congress Cataloging-in-Publication Data

Spirituality, health, and wholeness : an introductory guide for health care professionals / Siroj Sorajjakool, Henry Lamberton, editors.
    p. cm.
    Includes bibliographical references and index.
    ISBN 0-7890-1496-3 (hardcover : alk. paper) – ISBN 0-7890-1497-1 (pbk. : alk. paper)
    1. Medical care—Religious aspects. 2. Spirituality. I. Sorajjakool, Siroj. II. Lamberton, Henry.
BL65.M4S68 2004
201'.661—dc22

                2004000376

CONTENTS

ABOUT THE EDITORS

Siroj Sorajjakool, PhD, is Associate Professor of Religion and Program Director for the MA in Clinical Ministry for the Faculty of Religion as well as Research Associate for the Center for Spiritual Life and Wholeness for Loma Linda University. He has served as Section Co-Chair of Religion and Social Sciences for the American Academy of Religion, Western Region. He has authored two books, both published by The Haworth Press: *Wu Wei, Negativity, and Depression: The Principle of Non-Trying in the Practice of Pastoral Care* and *Child Prostitution in Thailand: Listening to Rahab.* He also has had articles published in the *Journal of Pastoral Care,* the *Journal of Religion and Health, Pastoral Psychology, Ministry Magazine, Dialogue,* and *Spectrum Magazine.*

Dr. Sorajjakool has pastored three churches in Thailand and served as Director of Thailand Adventist Seminary, Academic Dean for Mission College's Muak Lek Campus, and Associate Director for the Adventist Development and Relief Agency. He is currently a Fellow in the American Association of Pastoral Counselors and is a member of the American Academy of Religion, the Adventist Society for Religious Studies, the Society for Pastoral Theology, and the Adventist Chaplaincy Ministry. He received two awards from the Claremont School of Theology: The President's Award for Academic Excellence (1999) and the Willis & Dorothy Fisher Scholarship (1998).

Henry H. Lamberton, PsyD, is Associate Dean for Student Affairs at the Loma Linda School of Medicine. He is also Assistant Professor in the Department of Psychiatry and Associate Professor in the Faculty of Religion at Loma Linda University. He is a licensed clinical psychologist and continues to carry on a part-time clinical practice. Dr. Lamberton has worked as a hospital chaplain, a church pastor, and college and university religion teacher. He has published articles about the influence of the integration of cognition and emotion on physician-patient interaction; the development of moral reasoning in medical students; and the process of mentoring student physicians.

CONTRIBUTORS

Leigh Aveling, DMin, received his doctorate from Claremont School of Theology. His other academic training includes marriage and family therapy. He currently serves as director of chaplaincy at Loma Linda University Behavioral Medicine Center. He has served as a chaplain for eighteen years during which time he has worked with a variety of patients. Currently, he works with oncology and surgery patients along with their family members. In addition, Dr. Aveling works in an addictions unit with a focus on helping patients regain sobriety. Dr. Aveling also serves as Adjunct Assistant Professor on the faculty of religion at Loma Linda University.

Ethan Benore, MA, is a doctoral candidate in clinical psychology at Bowling Green State University. He is currently completing his internship in pediatric psychology at The Kennedy Krieger Institute/The Johns Hopkins University School of Medicine. His research interests include the psychology of religion, coping in children and families, and pediatric psychology.

Lee S. Berk, DrPH, is Adjunct Assistant Professor of Family Medicine, Susan Samueli Center for Complementary and Alternative Medicine, College of Medicine, University of California Irvine; Associate Clinical Professor, Health Promotion and Education, School of Public Health, Loma Linda University; and Adjunct Associate Research Professor of Pathology and Human Anatomy, School of Medicine, Loma Linda University.

Brenda Cole, PhD, is a licensed clinical psychologist and Assistant Professor at the University of Pittsburgh Cancer Institute (UPCI). For the past nine years she has conducted research on the role of spirituality and existential issues in the adjustment to chronic illnesses, including cancer and heart disease. She has conducted quasi-experimental and experimental studies of spiritually integrative interventions for these populations using longitudinal designs and has obtained grant support through private foundations to pursue this work. Dr. Cole has also written on related topics: defining the concepts of spirituality and religion, spiritual surrender as a paradoxical means to control, forgiveness, and the design of spiritually integrative interventions. Most recently she has developed and tested two scales to assess two aspects of spirituality within the process of coping with illness. One scale assesses spiritual coping using subscales that differentiate the emotion, problem, and meaning-focused aspects of coping. The other scale assesses spiritual well-being in the form of positive and negative affect experienced toward the sacred (God, Higher Power, etc.). Dr. Cole currently has a National Institutes of Health (NIH) grant pending to study the effects of a spiritually focused meditation program for people coping with metastatic melanoma.

Carla Gober, MS, MPH, is Assistant Professor in religious studies and associate director of the Center for Spiritual Life and Wholeness at Loma Linda University. She is currently on study leave at Emory University to pursue a PhD in religious studies with an emphasis in memory, illness, and ethnography. She completed a master of science in marriage and family counseling, and a master of arts in public health education from Loma Linda University. Before joining the faculty of religion, she coordinated the development of four hospital-based bereavement programs and functioned as the program counselor for a hospital-based peer support program in her role as spiritual nurse specialist.

James Greek, DMin, received his doctor of ministry from Fuller Theological Seminary. He currently serves as the director of the Chaplain Department at Loma Linda University Medical Center and Adjunct Assistant Professor of religion at Loma Linda University. Dr. Greek plays an active role in providing clinical training on spiritual care for medical students and residents at Loma Linda University Medical Center.

Kenneth I. Pargament, PhD, is currently Professor of psychology at Bowling Green State University in the clinical psychology PhD program. He has published extensively on the psychology of religion, stress, and coping. A fellow of the American Psychological Association and the American Psychological Society, Dr. Pargament is author of the book, *The Psychology of Religion and Coping: Theory, Research, Practice* and co-editor of the book, *Forgiveness: Theory, Research, and Practice.* He is past president of Division 36 (Psychology of Religion) of the American Psychological Association. Dr. Pargament consults with national and international health institutes, foundations, and universities.

Reginald A. Pulliam, MA, is a doctoral candidate in clinical psychology at Loma Linda University. His research interests are in the area of psychology and religion with an emphasis on the link between spirituality and cognitive/emotional integration as predictors of behavior. He is currently developing a God Schema Inventory to address cognitive/emotional integration relative to spiritual, physical, and psychological health outcomes.

Johnny Ramírez-Johnson, EdD, MA, graduated from Harvard University where he majored in cultural psychology using ethnography as his main research methodology for looking at the role religious ideology plays in a Hispanic community. Dr. Ramírez-Johnson currently serves as Professor of theology, psychology, and culture at Loma Linda University, Graduate School, and the faculty of religion. He is actively involved in research on the interplay of religion and health as well as cross-cultural aspects of religion. He has published articles in various journals including *American Behavioral Scientist* and *Journal of Research on Christian Education;* he has published *AVANCE: A Vision for a New Mañana* with Loma Linda University Press (2003). This book reports on the largest study ever conducted of any U.S. group of Hispanic churches.

Richard Rice, PhD, graduated from the University of Chicago Divinity School, with a dissertation on Charles Hartshorne's Concept of Natural Theology. His published writings include seven books, several chapters in anthologies, and a number of scholarly articles.

Dr. Rice's distinctive theological orientation is expressed in *The Openness of God: A Biblical Challenge to the Traditional Understanding of God.*

Bryn Seyle, MA, is a graduate of Loma Linda University in clinical ministry. She has been involved in a study on faith and illness and how meaning is constructed among breast cancer patients.

Acknowledgments

This project emerged from the teaching context itself. It derived from attempts of various individuals to bring sharper focus and attention to the concept of spiritual care. We wish, first of all, to thank students at Loma Linda University in various departments and programs who helped to clarify concepts and ideas through discussions and interactions on prayer, spirituality, spiritual care, and other related issues. Gerald Winslow, dean of the faculty of religion, has been most supportive in the pursuit of this project. Gayle Foster spent numerous hours going through this manuscript, engaging in conversations, contacting various individuals, and offering wonderful editorial insights. Kelvin Thompson, our research assistant, worked on formatting this manuscript.

We wish to thank various contributors for the time and wisdom shared; Dr. Richard Rice for his theological and biblical perspective on the meaning of wholeness; Dr. Lee Berk for his research on laughter as it relates to the immune system; Drs. Brenda Cole, Ethan Benore, and Kenneth Pargament for very thorough research on spirituality and coping with trauma; Bryn Seyle for her research on ways cancer patients construct meaning based on their struggles with illness; Dr. James Greek for his practical suggestions on the principles of spiritual care; Dr. Carla Gober for wonderful insights on ways we can provide spiritual care for the dying and bereaved; Dr. Johnny Ramírez-Johnson for his multicultural perspectives on spiritual care; Dr. Leigh Aveling for his clinical experience relating to the topic of difficult patients; and Reginald Pulliam for researching the literature relating to difficult patients.

Introduction:
The Resurgence of Interest
in Spirituality and Health

Henry H. Lamberton

Interest has grown among health care professionals and the public in the relationship between spirituality and health. Literature searches show a large increase, beginning in the late 1980s, in the number of research articles that address this topic. In 1995, Harvard Medical School's Department of Continuing Education and the Mind/Body Institute of Boston's Deaconess Hospital sponsored their first national conference on Spirituality and Healing in Medicine. The large attendance and interest resulted in a series of follow-up conferences held throughout the United States over several years. In 1997, the Association of American Medical Colleges and the National Institute for Healthcare Research[1] cosponsored their first conference for medical school educators on spirituality in the medical school curriculum. By 2001, over seventy of the 125 allopathic schools of medicine in the United States offered required or elective courses in spirituality and medicine compared with just one school in 1992 (Puchalski, 2001).

This resurgence of interest has, for understandable reasons, not been without controversy. Religion and healing have been integrally linked throughout most of recorded history. The role of healer, priest, shaman, or other religious practitioners were one and the same. But, particularly in the West, the separation of religion and science that came with the Enlightenment and freed scientists from the constraints of the church, helped to open the way for dramatic scientific advances in health care. Partly because of this history, some are uncomfortable with calls for a greater integration of the health sciences and religion. Others argue that the epistemologies of science and religion are so fundamentally different (even though both may be valid) that attempts to bring the two fields together only invite confusion. Others point to the violations of the ethical principle of patient autonomy that can occur if health care practitioners introduce religious topics or methods into the patient care arena. Still others are concerned that a tendency to "blame the sick for being ill" will develop if a patient's spiritual orientation is held up as a significant determinant of health.

Although these are important concerns, a number of countervailing influences have encouraged the renewed interest in spirituality and health. One of these is the significant body of research that demonstrates a relationship between religion, spirituality, and health.[2] Another is the increased emphasis on training professionals to develop an awareness of, and respect for, cultural diversity. A third influence is the recognition of the strength of religion and spirituality as cultural forces (Shafranske and Malony, 1996).

Undoubtedly, spirituality and religion play a significant role in the lives of many who seek care from health professionals. National poles show that nearly 95 percent of the U.S. population answer yes to the question, "Do you believe in God?" Eighty-eight percent report that they pray to God and 66 percent percent say they agree or mostly agree with the statement, "prayer is an important part of my daily life." About 75 percent say they believe in an afterlife and 40 percent report weekly attendance at a church or synagogue (Hodge, 1996). For many, religion provides a basis for making value judgments and assigning meaning to life experiences. Surveys indicate that a majority of patients would like their caregivers to talk with them about their spiritual concerns related to their illnesses (Miller and Thoresen, 2003).

Although few would disagree that religion and spirituality significantly influence the values and practices of individuals and societies, there is much less agreement about how to define religion and spirituality. Consensus shows that religion is, to use the language of researchers, a multidimensional construct, too diverse to be meaningfully reduced to a single variable (Hood et al., 1996). The same can be said if we substitute the word *spirituality* in place of religion. (More will be said about distinctions between religion and spirituality as follows). If we were to design a research project in which we surveyed a random sample from a large population group to determine whether those who say they believe in God have better health than those who say they do not, we would be unlikely to find significant differences. This is because the vast majority of our sample would say that they do believe in God and our question would not describe, for example, what they believe about God, the importance of their beliefs, or how their beliefs influence their attitudes and behaviors. We would need to look more closely at the phenomenon of belief and its variations to find whether it was helpful or detrimental for an individual's mental or physical health.

One well-known investigation of variations in religious experience was conducted by Gordon W. Allport. Allport (1950) was the first to distinguish between "intrinsic" and "extrinsic" orientations among religious adherents. Hood et al. (1996) summarize Allport's definitions of these two concepts as follows:

> Extrinsic religion is described as "strictly utilitarian: useful for the self in granting safety, social standing, solace and endorsement for one's chosen way of life." Intrinsic religion "regards faith as a supreme value in its own right. It is oriented toward a unification of being, takes seriously the commandment of brotherhood, and strives to transcend all self-centered needs. . . . A religious sentiment of this sort floods the whole life with motivation and meaning." (pp. 24, 25)

The intrinsic-extrinsic construct, which illustrates the approach of focusing on a specific dimension of spirituality and religion, has fostered considerable research. Koenig (1999), for example, studied the qualities of well-being and life satisfaction as they were self-reported by 836 elderly living in the Midwest. He found that intrinsic religiosity was a stronger predictor of these qualities than financial security or social status.

Among the more recent examples of research that have focused on a specific dimension of religion and spirituality is the work of Kenneth Pargament (1997) who has been a leader in investigating how people use spirituality to help cope with traumatic or stressful life events. He and his associates have identified styles of spiritual coping that correlate with positive, healthful outcomes and other spiritual coping styles that correlate with negative outcomes.

Rice (2002) provides another example of the multidimensional nature of religious experience in his description of three factors that support membership in a religious community. These are believing, behaving, and belonging. The first includes the beliefs individuals hold about God and/or religion as well as the relative strength or importance (saliency) of these beliefs in their experience. Behaving involves the way people express their religion or spirituality through their actions, including actions they avoid and those (e.g., prayer or a distinctive form of dress) they practice. The third involves the way faith leads to involvement in a community, such as a church or synagogue.

Many other examples could be given of the multidimensionality of religion and spirituality and the perspectives from which their effect on behavior and health can be studied (Hood et al., 1996; Koenig, McCullough, and Larson, 2001; Pargament et al., 1995). An understanding of this research is beneficial for health care professionals in a number of ways. First, research that documents the potential health benefits (both mental and physical) of religion and spirituality provides a rationale for offering spiritual care to patients who want it. Second, an awareness of the variety and complexity of religious experience helps the caregiver avoid premature or simplistic judgments about a patient's faith. Third, research that develops and tests models to explain how spiritual beliefs, attitudes, emotions, and behaviors interact and influence health can increase the practitioner's skill of observation in a clinical setting. Furthermore, knowledge of such research can help overcome the natural tendency to limit one's view of spiritual phenomena to what can be seen from the viewpoint of his or her own experience—whether that experience has been positive or negative.

We have not tried to carefully define the meaning of the terms *religion* and *spirituality* or to distinguish between them. One reason is the notable lack of consensus regarding their definitions. This lack of consensus exists whether one considers how these terms are used by psychologists or sociologists of religion, spiritual care providers (including clergy), the media, or the general public (Hodge, 1996; Pargament et al., 1995; Zinnbauer et al., 1997; Zinnbauer, Pargament, and Scott, 1999). This does not, however, mean that the definitions of *religion* and *spirituality* are completely fluid or ambiguous. Hill and Pargament (2003) note that the concept of the sacred is the defining characteristic of what religion and spirituality have reference to:

> Although any definition of a construct as religious and spiritual is limited and therefore debatable, . . . the sacred is what distinguishes religion and spirituality from other phenomena. It refers to those special objects or events set apart from the ordinary and thus deserving of veneration. The sacred includes concepts of

God, the divine, Ultimate Reality, and the transcendent, as well as any aspect of life that takes on extraordinary character by virtue of its association with or representation of such concepts (Pargament, 1999). The sacred is the common denominator of religious and spiritual life. It represents the most vital destination sought by the religious/spiritual person, and it is interwoven into the pathways many people take in life. (p. 65)

Another reason we have referred to religion and spirituality together is that most of the empirical research that has identified significant relationships between religion/spirituality and health has been conducted using the more objective variables (such as church attendance), that are traditionally associated with religion (Powel, Shahabi, and Thoresen, 2003).

The trend toward distinguishing spirituality from religion began in the mid-twentieth century, during the same period of time that the membership and influence of mainline denominations was declining and the influence of secularism was increasing. Disenchantment with institutionalized religion led many to view religion as an impediment to authentic personal spirituality. Historically, conceptions of religion included elements of an individual's search for what was sacred or ultimately purposeful (Zinnbauer et al., 1997). More recently, spirituality has become a term of reference for an individual's personal quest for, or subjective experience of, whatever is sacred or of transcendent meaning. Zinnbauer et al. (1997) note that assigning these personal elements to "spirituality" has resulted in a narrowing of the concept of religion to refer to what is formally structured or institutionally grounded. If we use this distinction[3] we would acknowledge that an individual could be (1) spiritual but not religious, (2) religious but not spiritual, (3) both religious and spiritual, or (4) neither religious or spiritual.

Zinnbauer et al. (1997) studied how the terms spirituality and religion were used among persons representing a wide variety of geographical, psychosocial, and religious and spiritual orientations. They found a significant distinction between the way the two terms were used. These uses were along the lines just noted. They also found that the terms were not fully independent. Their Roman Catholic sample (taken from a conservative church in a small community), nursing home patients, and students from a conservative Christian college made little or no distinction in the way they used these terms. Those making the greatest distinction between religion and spirituality were "New Age" followers, mental health workers, and nontraditional Episcopalians.

These considerations of definition highlight two practical points for health care professionals. One is the importance of noting which definitions and measures are used when evaluating studies of how religion and spirituality affect health. The other is that the meanings of *religiousness* and *spirituality* will vary significantly depending on who is using the terms.

We use the term spirituality in the book's title to clarify that its primary focus is on meeting spiritual needs of patients from a diversity of faith traditions as well as those who do not identify themselves with an established or organized faith tradition. Although spirituality and religion are often positive influences with well-documented benefits for mental and physical health, they frequently take on forms that are toxic or harmful. Health care professionals will encounter individuals whose prior experiences with religion/spirituality have been predominately negative. For this and other reasons, not all patients want to have their caregivers address religious or spiritual issues. The patient's autonomy should always be respected and a discussion of religious and spiritual issues should never be imposed.

Knowing when and how to address spiritual issues is an art that is developed through the application of knowledge, skill, perception, and an attitude of respect for the patient. This book is intended to assist the health care professional in learning this art. It is designed to be a practical guide for health care professionals when they encounter patients for whom illness creates a crisis of faith as well as those for whom it provides support. The authors of the following chapters have had extensive experience in the areas about which they write. Most of the authors come from the Judeo-Christian or Judaic tradition. But they identify principles that they and others have found to be important in working with patients from a wide diversity of spiritual traditions.

Some of the chapters address the importance of "caring for the caregiver," or of the way a caregiver's self-understanding influences his or her work with patients. Richard Rice's opening chapter provides a unique perspective on the spiritual significance of caring for physical illness by looking at the work of Jesus. This perspective becomes especially relevant when one considers the far-reaching influence of this historical figure on the establishment of hospitals and other health care institutions. Many of the words and metaphors that are part of the health care vocabulary are derived from the Christian tradition (Winslow, 1996).

Rice also outlines a theological/philosophical basis for spiritual care by providing a wholistic view of persons. The various dimensions we ascribe to personhood (physical, mental, emotional, social, spiritual, etc.) are differentiations of convenience, but we must never forget that persons are indivisible and that each dimension affects the others. Care for the whole person requires attention to all of the dimensions that make us human, including the spiritual dimension.

Throughout history, human experience has led people to understand that the mind and body affect each other. But it is only recently that the biological mechanisms of the mind-body connection have begun to be understood. Two bidirectional linkages between the brain and the rest of the body have been well established. These are the biochemical linkages through the hypothalamic-pituitary-adrenal axis and the linkages through the central nervous system. Lee Berk's discussion in Chapter 2 of research he and others have conducted on the affects of mirthful laughter on the immune system will be of interest for its description of the physiology of the mind-body connection as well as the benefits of humor.[4] Equally relevant and intriguing are the findings he and his colleagues have made about specific physiological benefits of positive expectations. "We believe that the 'biology of hope' that underlies recovery from many chronic disorders includes, in part, the synonyms *optimism, anticipation, expectation* of positive interventions and experiences" (p. 34). Surely one of the benefits of spiritual care is the hope that it provides.

In Chapter 3, Brenda Cole, Ethan Benore, and Kenneth Pargament summarize pertinent findings from the extensive research by Pargament and his associates on spirituality and coping. The chapter provides an excellent integration of research and practice that is of immediate relevance for health care professionals. It also gives an important foundation for Chapter 4, "Faith, Illness, and Meaning."

We have referred to the close association between spirituality and hope. However, serious illness or injury also bring loss, loss that will almost inevitably create, to a lesser or greater degree, a crisis of meaning. This is especially true when there is a loss of reliance or trust in a divine protector. In Chapter 4 Siroj Sorajjakool and Bryn Seyle describe the development in theological perspective that creates the possibility of a renewal of meaning and trust in times of loss.

"The underlying premise of spiritual care," James Greek writes in Chapter 5, "is that [in the midst of pain or loss] God still takes an interest in the plight of people. Although miraculous intervention may not take place, there is always the promise of presence, encouragement, and strength to face the future." Providing spiritual care requires an awareness that people are at different places in their spiritual development even though they might have comparable spiritual needs.

> Spiritual care is not standing at the end of the bed with a Bible like a televangelist, attempting to influence the patient into making a decision. Spiritual care is coming close to the heart of patients so we become aware of their burdens, both above and below the surface. (p. 105)

Greek provides twelve guidelines that provide a solid base for spiritual care. These include learning to "create a safe atmosphere. . . be aware of your surroundings. . . ask well chosen questions. . . mirror what you hear. . . and network (i.e., do not expect to be able to address all of a patient's emotional or spiritual concerns yourself)." While these guidelines are written from the perspective of Greek's work as a chaplain, they are worth the time for any caregiver to study and practice.

In Chapter 6, Carla Gober brings the perspective of a nurse and family therapist to the important subject of spiritual care for the dying and bereaved. She describes different types of losses and significant theories about how people move through loss, but notes that, "Providing good bereavement care is complicated." This is because of the variations among people, culture, genders, and the circumstances (varying from death that accompanies a protracted illness, a miscarriage, or a tragic accident) that bring loss. She joins the other authors in providing experiences from the patient care setting which illustrate the important principles discussed.

In Chapter 7, Johnny Ramírez-Johnson addresses issues of cultural diversity as they affect delivery and access to health care. This is a challenging topic. By definition, the subject of diversity resists the tendency to make meaningful generalizations, or look for "one-size-fits-all" solutions. Culturally competent spiritual care, as Ramírez-Johnson notes, requires a willingness to move outside of one's normal comfort zone.

Leigh Aveling, Siroj Sorajjakool, and Reginald Pulliam complete the book by addressing an area that inevitably challenges a caregiver's comfort zone. This is the challenge of working with difficult patients. These patients may include, to give a partial list, those that resist medical advice, or demonstrate hostility, impatience, excessive dependence or independence or exhibit inappropriate drug-seeking behavior. Working with difficult individuals is an inevitable part of a caregiver's experience. Providing spiritual care is not necessarily easy, nor is it simply a matter of technique. Overcoming the tendency to respond to anger with anger, or to dependence with avoidance, is evidence that an internal process of spiritual development has taken place within the caregiver. The results of this development are described as the "fruits of the spirit" in a classic statement by the apostle Paul. These fruits, he wrote, are "love, joy, peace, patience, kindness, goodness, faithfulness, gentleness, self-control" (Galatians 5: 22, 23).

The editors wish to thank each of the individuals who contributed to this book. Our own understandings have been enriched by the viewpoints and approaches that have been identified. Although points of view may not in all cases reflect views of the editors, a readiness to listen to a variety of perspectives and experiences is a fundamental part of what it means to give spiritual care.

NOTES

1. The National Institute for Healthcare Research has since been renamed the "International Center for the Integration of Health and Spirituality."

2. For a comprehensive review and discussion of this research, see Koenig, McCullough, and Larson (2001), *Handbook of Religion and Health;* and Koenig, H. G. (Ed.) (1998), *Handbook of Religion and Mental Health.*

3. Hill and Pargament (2003) note that while contrasting religion and spirituality may have some utility, there are several pitfalls to this approach researchers should be aware of: "First, the polarization of religion and spirituality into institutional and individual domains ignores the fact that all forms of spiritual expression unfold in a social context and that virtually all organized faith traditions are interested in the ordering of personal affairs," (Wuthnow, 1998, cited in Hill and Pargament, 2003). Second, implicit in the evolving definitions is the sense that spirituality is good and religion is bad; this simplistic perspective overlooks the potentially helpful and harmful sides of both religion and spirituality (Pargament, 2002, cited in Hill and Parga-

ment, 2003). Third, most people experience spirituality within an organized religious context and fail to see the distinction between these phenomena (Marler and Hadaway, 2002, cited in Hill and Pargament, 2003; Zinnbauer et al., 1997). Finally, the polarization of religion and spirituality may lead to needless duplication in concepts and measures. Current measures of religiousness cover a full range of individual and institutional domains. Purportedly new measures developed under the rubric of spirituality may in fact represent old wine in new wineskins" (pp. 64, 65).

4. Readers interested in further information about relationships between religiosity/spirituality and physiology are referred to the article: "Religiosity/Spirituality and Health: A Critical Review of the Evidence for Biological Pathways" by Seeman, Dubin, and Seeman, 2003. The article describes and evaluates studies of the physiological affects of zen, yoga, meditation/relaxation practices, and Judeo-Christian religious practices.

REFERENCES

Allport, G. W. (1950). *The individual and his religion: A psychological interpretation.* New York: Macmillan.

Hill, P. C. and Pargament, K. I. (2003). Advances in the conception and measurement of religion and spirituality: Implications for physical and mental health research. *American Psychologist,* 58(1), 64-74.

Hodge, D. (1996). Religion in America: The demographics of belief and affiliation. In E. P. Shafranske (Ed.), *Religion and the clinical practice of psychology* (pp. 21-41). Washington, DC: American Psychological Association.

Hood, R., Spilka, B., Hunsberger, B., and Gorsuch, R. (1996). *The psychology of religion: An empirical approach,* Second edition. New York: Guilford Press.

Koenig, H. G. (Ed.) (1998). *Handbook of religion and mental health.* San Diego: Academic Press.

Koenig, H. G. (1999). *The healing power of faith.* New York: Simon and Schuster.

Koenig, H. G., McCullough, M. E., and Larson, D. B. (Eds.) (2001). *Handbook of religion and health.* New York: Oxford University.

Miller, R. W. and Thoresen, C. E. (2003). Spirituality, religion and health: An emerging research field. *American Psychologist,* 58(1), 24-35.

Pargament, K. I. (1997). *The psychology of religion and coping: Theory, research, practice.* New York: Guilford Press.

Pargament, K. I., Sullivan, M. S., Balzer, W. K., Van Haitsma, K. S., and Raymark, P. H. (1995). The many meanings of religiousness: A policy capturing approach. *Journal of Personality,* 63(4), 953-983.

Powell, L. H., Shahabi, L., and Thoresen, C. E. (2003). Religion and spirituality: Linkages to physical health. *American Psychologist,* 58(1), 36-52.

Puchalski, C. M. (2001). Spirituality and health: The art of compassionate medicine. *Hospital Physician,* March.

Rice, R. (2002). *Believing, behaving, belonging: Finding new love for the church.* Roseville, CA: Association of Adventist Forums.

Seeman, T. E., Dubin, L. F., and Seeman, M. (2003). Religiosity/spirituality and health: A critical review of the evidence for biological pathways. *American Psychologist,* 58(1), 53-63.

Shafranske, E. P. and Malony, H. N. (1996). Religion and the clinical practice of psychology: A case for inclusion. In E. P. Shafranske (Ed.), *Religion and the clinical practice of psychology* (pp. 561-586). Washington, DC: American Psychological Association.

Winslow, G. R. (1996). Minding our language: Metaphors and biomedical ethics. In E. E. Shelp (Ed.), *Secular bioethics in theological perspective* (pp. 19-30). Dordrecht, Netherlands: Kluwer Academic Publishers.

Zinnbauer, B. J., Pargament, K. I., Cole, B., Rye, M. S., Butter, E. M., Belavich, T. G., Hipp, K. M., Scott, A. B., and Kadar, J. L. (1997). Religion and spirituality: Unfuzzying the fuzzy. *Journal for the Scientific Study of Religion,* 36(4), 549-564.

Zinnbauer, B., Pargament, K., and Scott, A. (1999). The emerging meanings of religiousness and spirituality: Problems and prospects. *Journal of Personality,* 67(6), 889-919.

PART I:
THEORY

Chapter 1

Toward a Theology of Wholeness: A Tentative Model of Whole Person Care

Richard Rice

OBJECTIVES

1. To conceptualize "ministryhealing" as a combination of health care and spirituality designed to address the multiple needs of patients.
2. To describe a model of wholeness and healing that incorporates an integrated view of humanity through four domains (spiritual, emotional, physical, and social).
3. To describe the process of caring *for* and caring *with* people as distinguished in the ministry of Jesus Christ, and its link to professionals working in health care settings.

INTRODUCTION

"Christianity measures the stature of man more highly and his virtue more severely than any alternative view" (Niebuhr, 1941, 1964, p. 161). Essentially, we are creatures in God's own image—made from the dust of the earth, yet capable of appreciating our creator and representing him in the world. As we actually exist, however, our condition is one of alienation and corruption. We are alienated from God, from others, from our environment, and ultimately from ourselves. We bear the damaging effects of sin in every aspect of our existence—physically, spiritually, emotionally, and socially. Every essential element of our humanity survives, but none in its original condition. To fulfill our destiny we need a solution to the wide-ranging problems that afflict us and lie beyond our capacity to solve. In a word, we need salvation. A Christian theology of healing, health, and wholeness thus regards the ultimate cause of illness as sin, the fundamental disorder that affects all of human existence, and views the attempt to overcome illness and restore life to its fullness as one aspect of God's saving work in the world.

The purpose of this discussion is to develop a model of healing and health care that reflects this complex vision of human existence. A model is a metaphor designed to provide a pattern for thinking and/or acting.[1] It serves a heuristic or explanatory purpose, and simplifies and sometimes distorts the reality it portrays in order to render it comprehensible. In a helpful discussion of the topic, Ian Barbour describes a model as "a symbolic representation of selected aspects of the behaviour of a complex system for particular purposes. It is an imaginative tool for ordering experience, rather than a description of the world" (Barbour, 1974, p. 6). The model of healing and health care proposed here draws from the central strand of Christian tradition, the Jesus story, and applies it to the complex view of humanity developed previously. A wholistic view of human existence involves a wholistic view of human sin, and this requires a wholistic concept of salvation.

The German language often brings words together to form expressions that generate new, more complex ideas. For example, *Heil,* meaning "salvation," joined with *Geschichte,* meaning "history," yields *Heils-geschichte,* a well-known theological term that can be translated as either "history of salvation" or "saving history." If we could do the same in English, a helpful expression for our purposes would be something like "ministryhealing." We could use it to express the notion that healing and ministry belong together—to show that healing is a form of ministry and ministry is a dimension of healing. This conjunction also suggests something stronger. It suggests that when ministry and healing come together they form a new and distinctive activity—something similar to each of them, to be sure, but more than just a combination of the two.

"Ministryhealing" is more than health care as conventionally understood—the treatment of physical disorders. It is also more than ministry as conventionally understood—attending to the "spiritual" or religious needs of people, apart from their physical and social needs. It is also more than an attempt to offer the two side by side as parallel forms of service. Ministryhealing is the attempt to integrate all the endeavors that address human needs in a comprehensive, coordinated program of human care. It presupposes that human beings are a complex reality comprising physical, mental, emotional, spiritual, and social dimensions, and arises from the conviction that we cannot deal with any of these dimensions without taking all of them into account. Accordingly, we must consider the whole person, or the person as a whole, whenever we address any particular problem or concern. Illness is a "whole person" problem. It involves human existence in all its dimensions. Every physical problem has emotional, spiritual, and social ramifications, and every emotional, spiritual, or social problem has a physical impact. Ministryhealing seeks to be a ministry that heals and a healing that ministers.

Ministryhealing presupposes the characteristic activities of a health sciences university. There are forms of wholistic treatment whose primary interest is nontraditional—alternative forms of medicine. Whatever their value, they are not our present concern. We are interested in the ways in which the various aspects of scientific medical care can be incorporated within an approach to healing that attends to the needs of the entire person as understood by Christian faith.

To develop a Christian theology of healing this chapter will take the route appropriate to a Christian theology of anything: the life and ministry of Jesus. In Jesus' life we see the model of ministryhealing, the ideal of whole person care. This is evident both in the care he gave *and* in the way he gave it. When Jesus ministered to people, he not only cared *for* the whole person, he cared *with* the whole person. Ministry was the central concern of his life; he poured his entire life into it. As the key text of the earliest gospel puts it, "The Son of Man came not to be served but to serve, and to give his life a ransom for many" (Mk 10:45). Accordingly, this chapter explores the ministryhealing of Jesus under two headings—care for the whole person and care with the whole person; it will show how each involves the essential dimensions of human life—physical, spiritual, emotional, and social.[2] The model for health care that Jesus' ministryhealing suggests will then be outlined.

MINISTRYHEALING IN THE LIFE OF JESUS

A model for this approach to integrated-integrative care can be found in the ministry of Jesus, who addressed concrete human needs across the entire scope of our existence. His concern for spiritual well-being comes most readily to mind, especially when we think of his various sermons and discussions. His concern for physical health is vivid, too, in his miraculous healings. But even a brief look at his ministry reveals that all aspects of human life concerned him.

The overarching theme of Jesus' preaching, according to the first three Gospels, was "the kingdom of God" or the "reign of God," as the original expression is more accurately translated (see Mk 1:15). Jesus announced the coming of God's kingdom. He urged people to prepare for its arrival. He told parables to illustrate its principles, and performed miracles to show what life in the kingdom is like. The miracles are obvious manifestations of his ministryhealing, and they bear a special relation to the kingdom of God.

As signs of the kingdom of God, Jesus' miracles assure us, first of all, that suffering is opposed to God's will. It does not belong in his universe. He seeks to eradicate it.

Jesus' miracles have what scholars call a "proleptic" quality. They are present manifestations of a future reality. Jesus' miracles show what life will be like when God's reign is fully realized. When God's plans for human beings are finally fulfilled, suffering will be a thing of the past. In God's kingdom, we will be free from all the destructive elements that dominate and intimidate us now. There will be no disease, death, or demonic possession. The world around us will be safe. We will be free from hunger and want. Nothing natural or supernatural will threaten our welfare.

Jesus' miracles show that God's kingdom is not only a reality yet to come, it is present now in significant ways as well. In fact, it is the ultimate basis for the world we live in. Jesus' miracles are windows on a deeper level of reality. They open our eyes to the ultimate order of things, and show that God is in charge now. Though blighted by sin, this is still "our Father's world."

Divine power is no less responsible for the food we eat daily than it was for the loaves and fishes that fed the 5,000 in Jesus' Galilean ministry. Divine power is no less responsible for our continued health and recovery from illness than it was for the people Jesus healed. His miracles show that "the ordinary is extraordinary." They reveal that God is at work in the world in unspectacular, unsensational ways. To quote Ellen White (1943, pp. 112-113),

> The Saviour in his miracles revealed the power that is continually at work in man's behalf, to sustain and to heal him. Through the agencies of nature, God is working, day by day, hour by hour, moment by moment, to keep us alive, to build up and restore us.

Like lenses that enable us to see in darkness, the miracles of Jesus open our eyes to the incessant workings of divine power that lie all around us.

Properly understood, then, the purpose of miracles is not to generate enthusiasm for more miracles. It is not to fuel the expectation that God will do what we want him to if we find the right formula, or ratchet our confidence up another notch or two. Instead, their purpose is to awaken us to the reality of God's presence in the world and the ways he constantly works to bless and benefit us. Miracles provide vivid demonstrations of the fact that God is always acting for our welfare.[3]

Jesus' miracles also reveal God's commitment to life in this world. The kingdom of God is not "otherwordly." People who enter the kingdom are not transported from this realm to another. The kingdom enters the world and transforms it. The apocalyptic vision of the new earth, with God's throne in the middle of the New Jerusalem, affirms the importance of human life to God. God dwells with humans, not by taking them away from this world to be with him, but by coming into the world to be with them. The kingdom of God affirms concrete human life in all its aspects.

With this general perspective in mind, let us explore the way in which Jesus' ministry embraces all dimensions of human existence.[4]

Jesus Cared for the Whole Person

Physical

Jesus' miracles affirm the value of physical health and provide a basis for endeavors to relieve suffering and heal the sick. Two-thirds of the miracles specifically described in the Gospels are miracles of healing—more if you count the three people Jesus raised from the dead and the demon-possessed who were ill as well. He cured blindness, deafness, leprosy, and paralysis. More accurately, he cured the blind, the deaf, the leprous, and the paralyzed, for his concern was directed primarily toward the victim, not the disease. Physical restoration was an essential part of Jesus' ministry.

We also see Jesus' concern for physical well-being in several of his so-called "nature miracles." He stilled a life-threatening storm on the Sea of Galilee, and on at least two occasions he fed the hungry crowds that followed him into the wilderness. The feeding of the 5,000, one of the few miracles mentioned in all four Gospels, illustrates the interrelation of the physical and spiritual in Jesus' thinking. It temporarily satisfied the hunger of a great many people, but the sermon Jesus preached shortly after, "The Bread of Life Discourse," connects this miraculous provision of physical food to the spiritual food that Jesus brings to human beings as "the bread from heaven." "I am the living bread that came down from heaven. Whoever eats of this bread will live forever; and the bread that I will give for the life of the world is my flesh" (Jn 6:51). So, our need for physical nourishment symbolizes our need for spiritual food, and Jesus Christ is the source of both.

Jesus' miracles affirm the importance of the physical. They also affirm the importance of what lies beyond the physical, and show that the two are intimately related. Man lives by bread, to be sure. But "man does not live by bread alone, but by every word that proceeds from the mouth of God" (Mt. 4:4). This brings us to the spiritual aspect of ministryhealing.

Spiritual

We tend to distinguish physical and spiritual maladies and assign them respectively to physicians and chaplains, or ministers. But Jesus dealt with spiritual and physical needs together. The Greek word for "heal," *sōzō,* also means "save," so it nicely expresses the view that spiritual and physical restoration are aspects of one comprehensive experience. When Jesus described his work as salvation, he no doubt saw it as including both physical and spiritual dimensions. In fact, on one occasion Jesus compared his work to that of a physician, suggesting that he envisioned his ministry as a whole as a ministry of healing, or "ministryhealing," to use our neologism.[5]

Jesus' entire ministry was directed toward spiritual ends, of course. Its primary objective was to restore human beings to a proper relationship with God. As we have seen, he announced that the kingdom of God was imminent, and saw himself as its personal representative. He invited people to enter the kingdom and described the various principles of "kingdom life" in numerous sermons and parables. He indicated that the relation of someone to the kingdom of God depended on his or her personal response to his ministry.

Although all of Jesus' miracles served a spiritual purpose as signs of the kingdom, a number of them made an explicit connection between the physical and spiritual dimensions of our existence. When four men brought a paralyzed friend to the house in Capernaum where Jesus was speaking and lowered him through the roof, Jesus' first words to him were, "Your sins are forgiven" (Mk 2:5). Only afterward did he say, "Rise, take up your pallet and go home" (2:11). There are several ways to interpret this sequence, but it shows that spiritual and physical restoration belong together, not merely in the sense that they are natural companions, but in the sense that they are integrally connected. Without spiritual health a person cannot be whole, whatever his or her physical condition may be.

Another miracle that brought physical and spiritual healing together involved the man born blind (Jn 9). Jesus restored his sight both physically and spiritually. As a result, he not only came to see for the first time, but recognized and believed in Jesus, the Son of man. Once again, the physical and spiritual were intimately connected, and the physical served as a symbol of the spiritual.

The close connection of physical and spiritual dimensions of human existence supports what some people call a "sacramental" view of reality—the concept that the physical world we inhabit is the bearer of transcendent meaning. One implication of this connection is the significance that attaches to the human body. A human body is more than a collection of cells, more than a physical object. It is the symbol of the person. We are incarnate beings; we exist in bodily form. But there is a mysterious "more" to our existence, and it is inextricably connected to the physical. Consequently, nothing physical is merely physical. What happens to us physically affects everything else about us—our mental outlook, our sense of identity, and ultimately our relation to God. The physical is the bearer of the spiritual. Physical features and actions convey meaning on the spiritual level, too.

The contact between the spiritual and the physical is perhaps most vivid in the various instances—half a dozen or so—in which Jesus cast out demons. Here again, we broach a topic that is complex and controversial,[6] but one message from Jesus' exorcisms is clear: spiritual powers have physical manifestations, and spiritual healing has physical consequences. In fact, healing means freedom from everything that dominates and depersonalizes us, and the restoration of every area of life where sin causes damage.

Emotional

The lines that separate the essential dimensions of human existence are not sharp—which is just what our wholistic view of the human requires. Whether ancient peoples envisioned human emotions as a discrete sphere of human existence is debatable.[7] So, we need to be cautious about talking about the emotions of biblical figures. From our perspective today, however, emotions are not only an important part of life, they may be the most important part. Indeed, for most people today, emotions have more to do with the quality of life than any other factor.

If we apply the category of emotions to scenes in the Gospels, it is evident that Jesus was highly sensitive to people's feelings. When he met people in great need, and healed their diseases, he took account of much more than their physical condition. Their feelings and attitudes were uppermost in his mind. A good example is his response to the woman who touched his garment in a desperate attempt to find relief from a hemorrhage. She was healed of her disease, but that was not enough for Jesus. He wanted to hear her story, too. So he listened while she poured out "the whole truth," as the Gospel puts it, and he called her "daughter" (Mk 5:24-34). Jesus also commended the woman for her faith, as he did others, such as the centurion who asked Jesus to heal his servant (Mt 8:10, Lk 7:9), and the Syrophoenician woman who begged him to heal her daughter (Mt 15:28).

Jesus showed great sensitivity to people's feelings, especially when they were the objects of neglect or scorn. He commended a poor widow for putting a mere pittance in the temple treasury (Mk 12:

41-44; Lk 21:1-4). He upheld Mary for choosing "the better part" when Martha complained that she was listening to him instead of helping her with household tasks (Lk 10:41-42). He praised the woman who washed his feet for doing a beautiful thing, and promised that the story of her deed would be told wherever the Gospel is preached in the whole world "in memory of her" (Mt 26:13; Mk 14:9). He comforted a woman harshly accused of adultery by assuring her, "Neither do I condemn you" (Jn 8:11). He was indignant when his disciples rebuked people for bringing their children to him (Mt 19:13-15; Mk 10:13-16; Lk 18:15-17). He embraced the "tax collectors and sinners" who came to him, over the grumbling of the Pharisees and scribes, and portrayed them in his greatest parables as valuable members of God's family.[8]

Jesus' ministryhealing included attending to the emotional needs of people. He was always sensitive to the way people felt, and took conspicuous, sometimes aggressive, measures to reassure them, particularly when they were vulnerable. He was strong in defending the weak, encouraging the fainthearted and lifting up the fallen. Conversely, he refused to sanction emotions of animosity and revenge. His most famous counsel on this appears in the Sermon on the Mount, where he urged his followers to love their enemies and pray for their persecutors (Mt 5:44). This attitude is evident throughout his life. On another occasion, he rebuked his furious disciples for wanting to call down fire from heaven to destroy some inhospitable Samaritans (Lk 9:52-55).

Jesus was also attentive to the emotional needs of his closest followers. When his disciples returned from a busy period of ministry, he encouraged them to come apart and rest awhile. He recognized their need for solitude to recover from the rigors of public life (Mk 6:31).

Social

To some scholars, Jesus was unique in offering the invitation to salvation to individual human beings, especially to individuals who lay outside the circle of religious respectability.[9] His open acceptance of sinners, women, and foreigners mystified his followers and scandalized his critics. He offered them places in the kingdom of God alongside Israelites of good and regular standing. In fact, he asserted they would enter the kingdom before these respectable people (Mt 21:31). We have looked at this form of ministryhealing in connection with Jesus' concern for people's emotions. But it applies more fundamentally to the social aspect of human life. Jesus did more than heal physical ailments, and his concern extended beyond individual human beings. His mission was to create a new community, to incorporate people within a fellowship whose members would exhibit the same love and support for one another that he displayed in his own life, who would reach out to embrace people from every nation and every station in life. In other words, Jesus envisioned the most inclusive community possible—a community open to everyone, to the entire world.

Consequently, the kingdom of God as Jesus described it reaches across every imaginable human barrier. It transcends all the differences that divide and separate people from one another—national, social, racial, cultural, political, economic, sexual, linguistic, and even moral. That's right—it ultimately bridges the widest of all chasms, the one that separates sinners and the sinned against, wrongdoers and their victims. Forgiveness obviously has a vertical dimension—it restores us to fellowship with God. But it has a horizontal dimension, too. It brings wrongdoers and their victims together and unites them in a fellowship of love. This is clearly the import of Jesus' comments on forgiveness, particularly his parable of the unforgiving servant (Mt 18:23-35). Its importance in the Christian scheme of things is clear from this request in the Lord's Prayer, "forgive us our debts as we forgive our debtors."

Given the fact that the kingdom of God was the central theme of Jesus' preaching, this is arguably the most important aspect of his ministry. The goal of his ministryhealing was the creation of community; the reconciliation of people to one another as well as to God.

We see the healing of communities in a number of Jesus' miracles, as well as his teachings on forgiveness. Each of the individuals he raised from the dead was restored to a bereaved family—Jairus' daughter, the son of the widow of Nain, and Lazarus of Bethany. Their physical restoration was a means of achieving social restoration. The same is true of other miracles. Jesus healed people of diseases that carried a strong social stigma, diseases that forced their victims to avoid society, to live apart from family and friends, and prevented them from participating in worship. This was particularly true of lepers and the woman who suffered from a hemorrhage. It was also true of the Gerasene demoniac who was banished to the tombs.

When Jesus healed these people of their various ailments, he restored them to their communities. He sent lepers to the priest to be examined (Mk 1:40-45). Once officially declared clean, they could return to their families. He pronounced a woman whose back he straightened a "daughter of Abraham," to remind those in the synagogue of her true identity (Lk 13:10-17). He sent the demoniac back to his friends and his home (Mk 5:19; Lk 8:39).

Jesus sometimes healed people in response to the faith of others. This is true of the centurion's servant, Jairus' little girl, the daughter of the Syrophoenician woman, an official's son, the paralytic in Capernaum, and the "epileptic" boy, whose father desperately sought Jesus' help. A person's illness is almost never an individual problem. It involves networks of relatives and friends. When someone is ill, everyone who cares deeply for that person is affected. Jesus acknowledged the social dimension of illness by responding to the faith of those who came to him, and by reestablishing the communities that death and illness had shattered.

Jesus' ministryhealing clearly involved care for the whole person—physically, spiritually, emotionally, and socially. In fact, there is no essential aspect of human life that his ministry did not touch.

Jesus Cared with the Whole Person

To a theological model of healing, the way Jesus cared for others is just as important as the others he cared for. He not only cared *for* the whole person, he also cared *with* the whole person. His concern for people was his consuming passion. It defined his existence. It affected every dimension of his life, just as it did the ones he helped. To appreciate all that ministryhealing involves, then, we need to review the way Jesus poured out his life in service.

Physical

We do not often think of Jesus giving of himself physically, but according to the Gospel accounts of his ministry, he did so frequently. When Jesus reached out to the sick, he did so literally. He customarily put his hands on those he healed (unless, of course, they were healed at a distance). He touched lepers, even though they were ritually "un-clean" (Mk 1:40-41). He touched Peter's mother-in-law, lifting her up by the hand, and her fever left her (Mt 8:15; Mk 1:31). He spat on the ground, made clay and put it on the eyes of the man born blind (Jn 9:6). He healed a deaf-mute by putting his fingers in the man's ears, then spitting and touching his tongue (Mk 7:31-35). He took children in his arms and blessed them, laying his hands on them (Mk 10:13-16). He washed his disciples' feet and wiped them with a towel (Jn 13:5). Jesus' willingness to touch people gave his care for them a concrete, palpable quality. Jesus did not love people in the ab-stract. He loved them as specific, individual, flesh and blood human beings. He cared for them as persons.

Jesus also allowed people to touch him. The crowds jostled him as he walked through Capernaum's narrow streets (Mk 5:24, 31). He praised the woman who bathed his feet, kissed them, anointed them with costly ointment, and wiped them with her hair. He accepted her devotion in the spirit in which she offered it, praised her for her faith, and assured her that her sins were forgiven (Lk 7:36-50; Jn 11:2). The most vivid demonstration of Jesus' submission to the care of others followed his crucifixion. His friends and followers prepared his body for burial and placed it in a tomb.

We see another aspect of Jesus' willingness to give physically in that he sometimes ministered to the point of exhaustion. Bone weary, he slept through a storm in the back of a fishing boat while his disci-ples battled the elements for their lives (Mk 4:35-41). On other occa-sions he grew hungry and thirsty.

There is a powerful symbolism in Jesus' physical manifestations of sympathy and love. His willingness to touch and be touched demon-strated that he cared for people in a concrete personal way, and he ac-cepted them, too. No one was too sick, too unclean, too ugly to re-ceive his touch.

Spiritual

Jesus' care for others was the central burden of his relationship to God. The Bible indicates that Jesus spent a good deal of time in prayer (Mk 1:35). In the best-known incident, his prayer in Geth-semane, he prayed for himself, of course. He pled with God to re-move the cup of suffering that lay before him. But he also prayed for others. In the great intercessory prayer of John 17, Jesus poured out his concern for his inner circle of followers. He prayed for their spiritual security and the success of their future mission in the world. There are indications that he prayed for people individually, too. When Simon Peter boasted of his loyalty, Jesus replied, "I have prayed for you that your own faith may not fail" (Lk 22:32).

The welfare and security of his disciples were uppermost in his mind. When Jesus was arrested, he asked his captors to let his companions go (Jn 18:8). During his crucifixion, in the throes of his final agony, he made provision for his mother's care (Jn 19:26-27). In the so-called "farewell discourses," the extent of Jesus' concern for others became vividly apparent. Jesus offered his followers his own fellowship with the Father. His highest joy was to bring them into the intimate circle of love that defined his own relationship with God. He wanted them to enjoy the same privileges he did (Jn 14:17).

Emotional

In the language of our day, we would describe Jesus as someone who was willing to be emotionally vulnerable. He opened himself to the feelings of other people, and he was equally generous in expressing his own feelings. Jesus was highly responsive to the people around him and deeply affected by their behavior. When a rich young man ran up to him, knelt down, and asked Jesus to help him find eternal life, Jesus looked on him and "loved him," according to one account of the incident (Mk 10:21).

On several occasions, according to the Gospels, Jesus was "moved with compassion" or "pity" when faced with human need—when he met a leper (Mk 1:41), when he witnessed the sorrow of a mother whose only son had died (Lk 7:13), and when he saw the crowds following him, "like sheep without a shepherd" (Mk 6:34).[10] The Greek word behind this expression is a blunt and forceful term, referring to the inner parts or organs of the body. It connotes deep-felt, spontaneous emotions that affect us viscerally, so to speak, as opposed to the "nobler affections like love and hate, courage and fear, joy and sorrow" (Koester, 1971, p. 549). These scenes of human suffering hit Jesus in the pit of his stomach. In a similar way, Jesus was deeply moved by the mourners as he neared the grave of his friend Lazarus, and burst into tears himself (Jn 11:35).

Jesus was also astonished and surprised at people's behavior. He marveled when people showed great faith, like the centurion (Mt 8:10), and when they showed little faith, as at Nazareth, his childhood home (Mk 6:6). We also sense that Jesus was sensitive to the way people responded to him, and deeply disappointed when they rejected him. There is a touching scene after his sermon in Capernaum when the multitudes, disillusioned with the dramatic claims he had made for himself, left him as readily as they had come not long before. He turned to his disciples and asked, "Do you also wish to go away?" (Jn 6:67).

Undoubtedly, the emotion we most readily associate with Jesus is love. This is most evident in his relationships with his disciples, his closest followers, and his innermost circle of friends. As the introductory verse to the passion story of the fourth Gospel puts it, "when Jesus knew that the hour had come to depart out of this world to the Father, having loved his own who were in the world, he loved them to the end" (Jn 13:1). "Loved to the end" may refer to the fact that Jesus loved his disciples to the very end of his life, which is certainly true. It may also indicate that Jesus showed the full extent of his love for them by taking the path that led to Calvary. If so, his actions bear witness to his words, "Greater love has no man than this, that a man lay down his life for his friends" (Jn 15:13).

Social

Jesus was generous with his company. He spent a great deal of time in public. He mingled with people freely. He shared his provisions with them, and accepted their hospitality in return. He ate with the in crowd, with Pharisees, and with social outcasts as well (Lk 7:36; Lk 15:1-2). In fact, Jesus was so social that his critics accused him of being "a glutton and a drunkard, a friend of tax collectors and sinners" (Mt 11:19; Lk 7:34). The Gospels show that Jesus could engage people from completely different social strata. John 3 records his conversation with Nicodemus, a Pharisee and member of the Sanhedrin, the highest Jewish council. John 4 records his conversation with a Samaritan woman who had a checkered sexual history. We cannot imagine a social situation that would bring Nicodemus and this woman together, yet Jesus was perfectly at ease with each of them.

Jesus lived his life in close association with other people. He gathered an inner circle of disciples around him and devoted a great deal of time to them. They were the beneficiaries of his most extensive teaching, so they in turn could minister to others (Mt 5:1). But Jesus reached beyond them as well. In fact, one of the central burdens of his ministry, as we have seen, was to establish a community that recognized no boundaries, a community open to every human being. To illustrate the nature of this community, the kingdom of God, he developed conspicuous associations with those least likely to be candidates for God's kingdom in the conventional thinking of the day.[11] He identified with the suffering. In the great parable of sheep and goats, the king identifies himself with the hungry and the thirsty, the stranger, the naked, the sick, and the imprisoned (Mt 25:37-40).

Jesus was so committed to offering others his companionship that he had no place to call his own. As he exclaimed on one occasion, "Foxes have holes, and the birds of the air have nests; but the Son of man has nowhere to lay his head" (Mt 8:20, Lk 9:58). He sacrificed all personal comfort and security so others could benefit from his ministry. Jesus affirmed human happiness. He attended feasts and celebrations, and he performed his first miracle at a wedding. Here his purpose was not to relieve someone of physical suffering, but to protect the groom from embarrassment and ensure the happiness of a new home.

When we look at the various dimensions of Jesus' own life, it is clear that he poured himself out in service and ministry. Every aspect of his person was devoted to others. Physically, spiritually, emotionally, and socially—Jesus drew on every facet of his life to bless and benefit others. It is no wonder that Christians have viewed his ministry as a costly sacrifice, and find a precedent for his life and work in the servant songs of Isaiah. He identified with the objects of his care so completely that he became one with them. He suffered in their suffering, and his suffering became the means of their salvation.

> He was despised and rejected by others; a man of suffering and acquainted with infirmity. . . . Surely he has borne our infirmities and carried our diseases; yet we accounted him stricken, struck down by God and afflicted. But he was wounded for our transgressions, crushed for our iniquities; upon him was the punishment that made us whole, and by his bruises we are healed. (Isa 53:3-5)

The ministryhealing Jesus demonstrated is impressive in both scope and intensity. There was no aspect of human existence that did not concern him, there was no one who lay outside the circle of his compassion, and there was no resource available to him that he did not invest in the attempt to meet people's complex and varied needs. He drew on the full range of his personal powers to meet the needs of others, and he emptied himself of these resources. When his ministry came to an end, he could have done nothing further to achieve the goals of his mission. He had explored all physical, mental, emotional, and spiritual resources available to him. His sacrifice was complete. When Jesus reached the end of his life, he had revealed "the full extent of his love" (Jn 13:1).

MINISTRYHEALING IN OUR LIVES

What theology of healing emerges from this account of Jesus' ministryhealing? What model for our healing endeavors does this theology suggest? It has implications for both care receivers and caregivers. It calls us to care for the whole person, and with the whole person.

According to the biblical view of human existence, human beings are creatures belonging to the complex biosphere of our planet, whose distinctive qualities endow them with unique dignity and power. Their misuse of these qualities has plunged them into terrible tragedy. The only creatures whose destiny lay within their own hands thwarted the purpose of their existence. But the Creator is also the Redeemer, and God is at work to overcome the consequences of sin and achieve his original purpose for humanity. God incorporates natural resources in this process, and ministryhealing is one way of participating in God's own work of salvation. From a theological standpoint, the health sciences are an extension of God's redemptive work in the world, a manifestation of his abiding commitment to human welfare, and an example of his providential use of human abilities and energies to achieve his purposes.

Caring for the Whole Person

Ministryhealing involves a vision of comprehensive health care in a number of important ways. First, it is comprehensive in the sense that it extends to all human beings. All should have the medical resources they need to meet life's physical challenges. Those who participate in the ministryhealing of Jesus will recognize that no one is undeserving of health care. They will find ways to extend the benefits of modern medicine to everyone who would benefit from them.

Second, the health care that ministryhealing envisions is comprehensive in the sense that it extends to the entire life experience. What assistance is needed at the beginning of life? What is needed at the end? Health caregivers engaged in ministryhealing view disease and death as enemies, yet they recognize that we live in a world in which salvation is not yet a full reality. Certain conditions and situations force us to recognize that complete healing will not take place until the kingdom of God becomes a concrete reality in the world. Ministryhealing acknowledges the value of a human being whose problems surpass the limits of human nature and the limits of human knowledge. No one involved in ministryhealing will "check out" when a person's physical problems pass the point where there is any known solution.

Third, the health care that ministryhealing envisions is comprehensive because it affirms the full humanity of each human being. No human being is complete, in the sense of being everything God intends him or her to be. In some cases this incompleteness is more obvious and apparently more drastic than in others. But Jesus treated everyone he met as a person of infinite value, a child of God, and a potential citizen of the kingdom of heaven. No one was worthless or dispensable, contrary to popular opinion. In fact, Jesus identified himself with some pathetic examples of human misery. So also, ministryhealing addresses the needs of the most desperate members of the human family.

Finally, the health care that ministryhealing envisions is comprehensive because it addresses all the dimensions of human existence, all the things that make us human—physical, spiritual, emotional, and social. It recognizes that human wholeness requires health in all these areas.

Physical needs are the most obvious and often the most pressing, but they are seldom isolated from other needs. People with physical problems almost always have spiritual, emotional, and social needs as well.

Spiritual needs may not seem as pressing at times as physical ones, but they are more fundamental, so ministryhealing makes spiritual health its highest priority. It envisions each human being as a child of God and looks for ways to bring people to a knowledge of God's love for them and their identity as God's children. From the perspective of ministryhealing, sick people are not sophisticated machines that need repair, but persons that need care.

Every sick person experiences emotional as well as physical distress. Ministryhealing must take this into account. Whatever people's physical condition, the spiritual identity and potential of each person entitles them to be treated with respect and dignity. If we cannot assure them that all is well physically, we can reassure them of their infinite value to God.

Human beings are social; we live in relationships. Ministryhealing takes note of the "significant others" in the life of each sufferer. This is why it is important to have caregivers who have special skills in restoring relationships.

Ministryhealing is a multifaceted endeavor that requires caregivers to cultivate a sensitivity to the full spectrum of human needs and develop a variety of abilities to deal with them. When possible, ministryhealing brings together people who have a diversity of complementary skills and a determination to coordinate their application to the needs of the people they serve.

Caring with the Whole Person

Ministryhealing is not a business, career, or profession. It is fundamentally a calling—a calling to serve. To participate in Jesus' saving ministry to this world, caregivers draw on all their human resources.

Obviously, it takes physical strength and stamina to meet pressing human needs over time, especially when many of them are critical. So, ministryhealing can be a costly activity. A more specific physical resource that appears in the ministry of Jesus is the power of touch. A touch has a personalizing effect. It reassures the care receiver that he or she is not just a condition, a case, or a chart, but someone whose humanity and individuality deserve to be recognized and affirmed. Other physical gestures that "connect" with care receivers can contribute to the healing process as well, such as taking a position close to the patient, speaking directly to, and looking at the patient.

Ministryhealing is essentially a spiritual activity. It consists of participating in God's own redemptive work in the world. For this reason, those who participate in such ministry draw strength from a sense of God's presence in their lives. They consciously remind themselves that they are God's agents in the world, that they share with Jesus the work of relieving human suffering. Should they communicate their religious concerns for those who are sick in an explicit way? Such questions often provoke heated replies. Some people feel that it is manipulative or coercive for caregivers to broach religious issues with their patients. On the other hand, people have spiritual needs, and often become aware of them when they suffer, and caregivers can provide a valuable resource at that time. The crucial question is how to respect a person's religious integrity and emotional vulnerability as we address their spiritual needs. This calls for great wisdom and skill.

To what extent should caregivers commit themselves emotionally to the objects of their concern? This is a perennial question, with no simple answer. But there is a growing recognition that emotion has an important role to play in the practice of medicine.[12] That kind of care cannot effectively deal with emotional needs without drawing on emotional resources. Surely a caregiver who refused to respond emotionally to a person in need would be a contradiction in terms. For how could such a person provide "care" in any significant way? On the other hand, how could a person who spends herself or himself unstintingly in caring for others avoid running out of emotional energy long before his or her responsibilities are fulfilled? Perhaps the solution is not to keep from spending oneself emotionally, but to find ways of replenishing one's emotional resources.

When it comes to the social aspect of caring, ministryhealing brings caregivers and care receivers together to form a community, or fellowship. To achieve healing and wholeness, they must work together. Ministryhealing recognizes that caregivers and receivers are united by a common illness. All of us are afflicted by sin,[13] and all of us need help from the same source. Science does not heal people, not in the full sense of the word. More accurately, it is the Lord who heals people, and the human role is to learn how to cooperate with him. Caregivers and care receivers do not stand in a hierarchical relationship, where one directs or orders another. Instead, the community of caregivers includes care receivers themselves and unites their efforts in seeking to restore health. The ultimate goal of ministryhealing is spiritual community, and it sees the healing community as an avenue to this end.

GUIDED QUESTIONS

1. What view of the human person and what view of human health lies behind your concept of healing?
2. Do you believe that different forms of health care operate with different models of health and healing?
3. How will cultural and economic factors in a given society affect the sort of healing its people seek and the sort of health care made available to them?
4. How would a commitment to "ministryhealing" affect the sort of health care we provide people?
5. What are the essential dimensions of human existence? How did Jesus minister to each of them?
6. What model(s) of healing does the ministry of Jesus suggest?

NOTES

1. Metaphors are pervasive in human speech; this is one of the indications that we are incarnate beings. We are embedded and embodied within a material world, and our mental life draws on this physical orientation to form the basic framework of our thought. Because our thinking is essentially metaphorical, our seeing is always "seeing as." We instinctively view things, and understand them, in relation to other things. One anthropologist attributes the origin of religion to this inherent tendency to see things *as* something else (Stewart Guthrie, *Faces in the Clouds: A New Theory of Religion,* 1993). Metaphors operate on virtually every level of life. We learn by making comparisons, and instinctively express ourselves by describing one thing in terms of another. Sportscasters are forever describing one sport with expressions derived from another. A boxer who knocks out an opponent in the final round "hits a grand slam in the bottom of the ninth." A baseball player who hits a grand slam with two out in the ninth inning "delivers a last-minute knockout." When someone asked golfing great Bobby Jones if he felt sad about his debilitating spinal condition, he replied, "Remember, you play the ball as it lies" *(Newsweek,* October 25, 1999, p. 52). Some metaphors are invented—poets in particular are good at this—but most of them arise spontaneously. The prevalence of metaphors is also evident in the sweeping influence of paradigms. Paradigms are large-scale models that exert great influence. They characterize the way large groups of people, entire professions, historical epochs, or even whole cultures, characteristically look at things. Thomas Kuhn's

(1970) book on scientific revolutions is the classic discussion of paradigms. In fact, ever since its publication, the word "paradigm" has itself become a paradigm for large-scale, epochal perspectives. Though they do not use the word "paradigm," Judith Allen Shelly and Arlene B. Miller (1999) apply the idea when they describe nursing and medicine as "two distinct professions with very different histories. Western medicine developed out of a Greek, and later Cartesian, body-mind dualism that viewed the body as object. The role of the nurse, however, grew out of a Christian understanding of the human person as created in the image of God and viewed the body as a living unity and the 'temple of the Holy Spirit' (1 Cor 3:16). Medicine has traditionally focused on the scientific dimension of the human body, relegating the spiritual and psychosocial dimensions to religion and psychology. The uniqueness of nursing is its emphasis on caring for the whole person as embodied" (p. 16).

2. It is always risky to list different aspects of human existence, because it inevitably creates the impression that human beings are made up of various parts or pieces. This is obviously opposed to the view of humanity proposed here. Every facet of human life relates to every other, and none of them is separable from the whole. For purposes of discussion, however, a provisional distinction must be made.

3. We are concerned here with the theology of healing Jesus' miracles suggest. The philosophical literature dealing with miracles is vast, of course, and tends to focus on the question of whether extraordinary or "supernatural" events are metaphysically possible. The issue is important, but it has limited relevance to our interests here

4. Any list of human qualities, or enumeration of life's dimensions, will seem arbitrary. In addition to the four that figure prominently in this discussion, there are others that deserve attention, too, such as the intellectual, psychological, cultural, and environmental facets of our lives, and the developmental nature of everything about us. Human beings are always in process, always on the way. We are never everything that we are meant to be. We touch on some of these neglected aspects of life—emotional and spiritual facets bear directly on what we think of as intellectual and psychological—but others, such as the cultural and ecological, are not involved. In view of their unavoidable limitations, these comments should be viewed primarily as suggestive. A great deal more could be said about the important topic before us. I am confident that this general approach is potentially comprehensive. There is no aspect of human life that Jesus' ministryhealing did not, and does not, touch and transform.

5. "Those who are well have no need of a physician, but those who are sick." Mt 9:12.

6. Some people are inclined to view the Gospel accounts of "demon possession" as archaic descriptions of what we diagnose as psychiatric disorders today. Others see them as indications that human beings are locked in "spiritual warfare" with evil agents from another order of reality, who invade human minds and bodies and cause great suffering.

7. Krister Stendahl (1963) raises serious questions about "psychological" interpretations of Paul's writings.

8. See the parables of the lost sheep, the lost coin, the prodigal son (Lk 15).

9. In fact, there are even those who suggest that it was Jesus' openness to the outcast and downtrodden that ultimately accounted for his execution.

10. The same expression appears in Jesus' parables, which describe the feelings of the father for his wayward son and the response of the good Samaritan to the wounded traveler on the Jericho road in Lk 15:10; 10:33.

11. The citizens of the kingdom Jesus describes in the Beatitudes include a surprising group of people—the poor, the meek, those who mourn, the merciful, the persecuted, the hungry and thirsty, etc.—not the sort most people would expect to build up a kingdom of any significance (Mt 5:3-13).

12. See the discussion in *Empathy and the Practice of Medicine* (Spiro et al., 1993).

13. George Khushf (1995) makes this point forcefully by describing illness as "general revelation," as "revelatory of the human condition in general," and as "a manifestation of the structure of sin" (pp. 108-109).

REFERENCES

Barbour, I. G. (1974). *Myths, models and paradigms: A comparative study in science and religion.* New York: Harper and Row.

Guthrie, S. (1993). *Faces in the clouds: A new theory of religion.* New York: Oxford University Press.

Khushf, G. (1995). Illness, the problem of evil, and the analogical structure of healing: On the difference Christianity makes in bioethics. *Christian Bioethics,* 1(1), 108-109.

Koester, H. (1971). In G. Friedrich (Ed.), trans. by G. W. Bromily, *Theological dictionary of the New Testament* (Vol. VII, p. 549). Grand Rapids, MI: Eerdmans.

Kuhn, T. (1970). *The structure of scientific revolutions,* Second edition. Chicago: University of Chicago Press.

Shelly, J. A. and Miller, A. B. (1999). *Called to care: A Christian theology of nursing.* Downers Grove, IL: InterVarsity.

Spiro, H. M., McCrea Curnen, M. G., Peschel, E., and St. James, D. (Eds.) (1993). *Empathy and the practice of medicine: Beyond pills and the scalpel.* New Haven, CT: Yale University Press.

_____ *Newsweek,* October 25, p. 52. (1999).

Stendahl, K. (1963). The apostle Paul and the introspective conscience of the West. *Harvard Theological Review,* 56, 199-215.

White, E. G. (1943). *Ministry of healing.* Washington, DC: Review and Herald Publishing Association.

Chapter 2

Mind, Body, Spirit: Exploring the Mind, Body, and Spirit Connection Through Research on Mirthful Laughter

Lee S. Berk

People tell me not to offer hope unless I know it to be real, but I don't have the power not to respond to an outstretched hand.

Norman Cousins

Belief affects Biology.

Norman Cousins

There is no medicine like hope, no incentive so great, and no tonic so powerful as expectation of something tomorrow.

O. S. Maden

Totally without hope one cannot live. To live without hope is to cease to live. Hell is hopelessness. It is no accident that above the entrance to Dante's hell is the inscription: "Leave behind all hope, you who enter here."

Fyodor Dostoyevsky

OBJECTIVES

1. To discuss the interrelation of physical, mental, and emotional domains as applied to wholeness principles in health care.
2. To describe the physiological impacts of humor on the immune system.
3. To describe the physiological impacts of hope and humor on mood and the neuroendocrine hormones.
4. To discuss the importance of incorporating wholeness principles into the practice of medicine.

INTRODUCTION

"Imagine a prescription that reads: *One Abbott and Costello, followed by doses of Charlie Chaplin, W. C. Fields, and Buster Keaton. Wash down with Marx Brothers. Repeat as necessary. Call me in the morning*" (Rayl, 2000, p.18).

Can the benefits of humor protect against or possibly even help in the healing process from a disease? Can we laugh ourselves toward health? Can the anticipation of positive events and behaviors benefit our health? These are the questions we want to consider. This chapter starts with a brief history of how research on the effects of humor and the associated mirthful laughter on the immune system began and then summarizes results of several such studies in this area. Viewed from a larger perspective, the research described in this chapter has made a significant contribution to our understanding of the interrelationship of mind, body, and spirit.

BACKGROUND OF THE STUDIES

"Can humor cause a positive physiological impact? Could the gags, quips, and shtick of such legends as Charlie Chaplin, Bud Abbott and Lou Costello, and the Marx Brothers, or some of today's comedians, really be medicinal?" asks Rayl (2000, p. 1).

During the last couple of decades—since the best-selling author Norman Cousins made headlines by "laughing" himself well— researchers have been working to uncover the physiological impact of laughter at the cellular and neurochemical level. By all indications, the eons-old notion is grinning and bearing out. (Rayl, 2000, p. 1)

Back in the mid 1980s I was approached by Norman Cousins[1] to do research on the relationship between laughter and health. The purpose was to investigate if there was empirical support for the theory that laughter facilitated the healing process. Our research team was given research funds to initiate studies. The first study investigated whether laughter had an impact on the stress hormones of the neuro-endocrine system. A number of medical students were asked to watch a video, *Gallagher—Over Your Head,* by the comedian Gallagher, and blood samples were taken. We learned that the humor associated with mirthful laughter can change and even reduce detrimental stress hormone levels in the peripheral blood. It was an exciting discovery to realize that humor could have such direct and measurable effects on human psychobiological functioning (Berk, Tan, Fry, et al., 1989).

Other researchers interested in the topic of laughter and medicine are Margaret Stuber, professor of psychiatry and behavioral science at UCLA, and Lonnie Zeltzer, director of the Pediatric Pain Program at Mattel Children's Hospital. Their five-year research program ("Rx Laughter") explored the impact of humor on the immune systems of dozens of healthy children and children with life-threatening diseases. According to Zeltzer:

> If you're laughing, you feel better in general. And since it elevates your mood, it should do something physically in your body to create that feeling of well-being. I think we're going to learn that exposing yourself to humor in life will not only change mood and reduce stress hormones but also influence serotonin levels, which are involved in the pain-control system. That would mean laughter could have an effect on chronic pain over time and enhance immunoreactivity, as well as help with depression and sleep and anxiety disorders. (cited by Rayl, 2000, p. 16)

Stuber and Zeltzer studied direct physiological responses of the autonomic nervous system by observing heart rates, blood pressure, and stress hormones and other hormones, neurotransmitters, and natural killer cells.

Peter Derks (Derks et al., 1997), another researcher interested in the role of humor in healing, and his colleagues at the College of William and Mary, did a study on the relationship between brain activity and humor using EEG topographical brain mapping. "They found that laughter affects substantial and significantly unique electrical activity, and that the whole brain is involved" (Rayl, 2000, p. 18).

"A merry heart doeth good like a medicine, but a broken spirit dries the bone" (Proverbs 17:22). Western society is accustomed to popping pills to kill pain and lift moods. But if "a merry heart doeth good like a medicine," can we laugh to kill pain and smile to lift moods? Perhaps, suggests Zeltzer, Rx Laughter's coprincipal investigator. "Maybe the prescription will include finding what the patient's favorite funny program is, prescribing it, and then looking at the impact on both symptoms and physiology" (Rayl, 2000, p. 18).

HUMOR AND THE NEUROENDOCRINE AND IMMUNE SYSTEMS

A number of studies have been conducted to ascertain the role of mirthful laughter and its impact on stress hormones and immune system components, such as Berk and Tan (1988a,b, 1995; Berk, Tan, Napier, et al., 1989); Berk, Tan, and Fry (1993); Berk et al. (2001); and Berk, Tan, Fry, et al. (1989).

RESEARCH FINDINGS

Findings from these research studies may be broadly summarized as follows:

1. *Increase in activated T cells:* Our bodies contain many T cells that are not turned on. They are just there waiting to be told to do something. Through our experiments we have found that people who are exposed to mirthful laughter have sufficient physiologi-

cal and chemical changes to activate these T cells. When these T cells are activated, it turns up the immune system and gets it ready to combat something foreign or function more effectively. Exercise has the same impact. People who exercise moderately seem to have a lower rate of cardiovascular disease, infections, and cancers.

2. *T Cells with helper/suppressor receptors:* Each cell in the human body has numerous receptors that bind chemicals such as neurotransmitters, hormones, or other modulators such as cytokines. The cell changes its metabolic activity as a consequence of these chemicals binding their specific receptor. These same chemicals can also bind to the receptors on T helper/suppressor immune cells. We discovered from our studies that there is an increase in the immune T cells with helper/suppressor receptors. This suggests that mirthful laughter may be capable of effecting the metabolic activity of these types of immune cells.

3. *Increase in the numbers and activity of natural killer cells:* Natural killer cells are immune cells that seek out virally infected cells and some types of cancer cells. These immune cells seek out the infected or cancer cells and attempt to destroy/kill them. Research findings measured an increase in the numbers of natural killer cells for subjects who experienced mirthful laughter, while there was no increase in the number of natural killer cells in the subjects that did not experience laughter. In addition, research also showed an increase in the activity of the natural killer cells. It is amazing that a "simple behavior" such as mirthful laughter can modulate and effect natural killer cells.

4. *Gamma interferon:* Gamma interferon is a type of chemical called a cytokine that is produced by the cellular arm, Th1, of the immune system. It is one of the substances produced by the immune system that communicates with other immune cells by attaching to the other cells' receptor. These Th1 cytokines play a significant role in activating lymphocyte and cytolytic functions associated with effective antitumor defense mechanisms. Research showed that gamma interferon is increased in association with the mirthful laughter experience.

ANTICIPATION OF POSITIVE HUMOR/MIRTHFUL LAUGHTER EXPERIENCES: A METAPHOR FOR THE SPIRIT OF HOPE

Subsequent to our original research on the effects of laughter on the immune system we studied how the mere anticipation or expectation of positive humor/mirthful laughter experiences brings about changes in a person's mood states and stress hormones. We believe these findings relate to the concept of hope and that they may give us some insight into the psychobiological mechanisms underlying the positive benefits of hope. Our research in this area was peer reviewed and presented at the Society for Neurosciences Annual Meetings in San Diego, California, November 2001 (Berk, Felten, and Westengard, 2001); Orlando, Florida, November 2002 (Berk et al., 2002); and at the American Public Health Association's Annual meeting in San Francisco, California, November 2002. An overview of the findings presented is described as follows.

Anticipation and Mood

Previous research has demonstrated that viewing of a self-selected humorous video for one hour can ameliorate many of the physiological effects of distress. Many forms of chronic stress result in suppressed immune responses, particularly those related to antiviral and antitumor defenses. These diminished immune responses appear to be the result of increased secretion of stress hormones such as cortisol and epinephrine. Mirthful laughter diminishes the secretion of cortisol and epinephrine, while enhancing the antiviral and antitumor immune reactivity. In addition, mirthful laughter enhances the secretion of growth hormone, an enhancer of these same key immune responses (Berk et al., 2001). Some biological effects of a single one-hour session of viewing a humorous video can last from twelve to twenty-four hours. Other studies of daily thirty-minute exposure to such humor/laughter videos have shown profound and long-lasting changes such as decreased heart rate, blood pressure, amount of medications needed, and few recurrences of heart attacks through the year of the study (Tan et al., 1997).

Research from these new studies demonstrates that anticipation/ expectation of a one-hour experience of mirthful laughter, such as viewing a humorous video, evokes a significant decrease in negative mood states and an increase in positive mood state up to two to three days prior to the actual viewing of the video.

In this study we administered the Profile of Mood States (POMS), an instrument that measures changes in tension, depression, anger, vigor, fatigue, and confusion. It was administered to ten fasting male subjects (mean age twenty-seven years) at time points two to three days before, fifteen minutes before, and immediately following, the viewing of a self-selected sixty-minute video. The POMS scores in each of the six areas were charted longitudinally and compared with published standardized test norms for the POMS. Table 2.1 shows the relative percentage decreases or increases in mood states.

Test subjects demonstrated a progressive pattern of significant decreases in depression, tension, fatigue, confusion, and anger (significant at a level of $p < 0.001$) and a significant increase in vigor (significant at a level of $p < 0.01$). Changes in mood states *began two to three days prior* to the viewing of the humorous video, and continued through and after the one-hour laughter intervention. This positive pattern of altered mood states represents a "eustress" profile that is counter/opposite to that provoked by classical stress (distress).

In conclusion, this study demonstrates that anticipation/expectation of humor can initiate changes in mood state prior to the actual experience itself.

It was hypothesized that the same anticipatory behavior or positive expectation that led to "better" mood states also would lead to the associated stress hormone changes (neuroendocrine mediators), again prior to viewing the humorous video.

Anticipation and Hormones

Another study on the effects of anticipation/expectation demonstrated that looking forward ("hopeful") to a positive experience, such as viewing a desired self-selected humorous video, evoked significant decreases in detrimental stress hormones and increases in a beneficial hormone and endorphins prior to the actual viewing. These findings and observations provide new insights into the understand-

TABLE 2.1. POMS Measurements for Six Areas

Mood States	Relative Percent Change from Test Norms		
	Two Days Before the Humor	Fifteen Minutes Before the Humor	After the Humor
Tension	−9	−35**	−61***
Depression	−51*	−91***	−98***
Anger	−19	−90***	−98***
Vigor	+12	+9	+37**
Fatigue	−15	−63**	−87***
Confusion	−36**	−63***	−75***

*p < .05   **p <. 01   ***p <. 001

ing of the psychobiology of the concept of positive anticipation, expectation, and hope.

In the second study half the subjects were informed two to three days prior to the humor intervention that they were in the "subjects in group," the experimental laughter group (watching the upcoming humorous video), and the other half were informed that they would be in the control group (not going to be watching the upcoming humorous video). More specifically, we studied sixteen healthy fasting male subjects for changes in β-endorphin, growth hormone, cortisol, epinephrine, dopac, prolactin, and norepinephrine in a eustress humor/laughter experiment. Two to three days prior to the intervention subjects were notified of their random group assignment. Blood was drawn before intervention, four times during, and three times post. Trend analysis showed a progressive pattern of eustress change with significant baseline decrease before the humor video in cortisol, epinephrine, and dopac and increase for β-endorphin and growth hormone (p < 0.01). No significant change was noted for prolactin and norepinephrine. We suggest that the anticipation, prior to the experience, of a positive humor/laughter eustress event initiated changes in neuroendocrine hormones (see Table 2.2) prior to the intervention. This would appear to be concomitant with our previous study on parallel mood state changes.

TABLE 2.2. Baseline Anticipation Summary Statistics for the Control and Experimental Groups for the Seven Stress Hormones and Endorphins

Stress Hormones	Group	Mean	Percent Difference
		Baseline Anticipation	
Cortisol (nMoles/L)	Experimental	240	
	Control	390	−39.0*
Beta-Endorphin (pMoles/L)	Experimental	14.8	
	Control	11.3	+27.0*
Growth Hormone (uG/L)	Experimental	9.2	
	Control	1.2	+87.0*
Prolactin (uG/L)	Experimental	6.4	
	Control	6.6	−3.0
Dopca (nMoles/L)	Experimental	14.11	
	Control	22.65	−38.0*
Epinephrine (pMoles/L)	Experimental	380	
	Control	1250	−70.0*
Norepinephrine (nMoles/L)	Experimental	2.14	
	Control	2	+6.5

*$p < 0.01$ statistical significance

We believe that support in the recovery from illness includes, in part, behaviors that represent *optimism, anticipation, expectation* of positive interventions and experiences—and may indeed constitute a real "biology in *hope*." If complementary and integrative interventions/adjunctive therapies, directed toward wellness and recovery from chronic diseases, can incorporate positive expectation or anticipatory experiences and behaviors—"hope," the resultant changes not only (1) contribute to beneficial positive mood state changes; but also, (2) modify important biological/chemical stress hormone and neuropeptide mediators that optimize immune responses; (3) diminish stress-related molecules and inflammatory mediators; and in total (4) contribute to the holistic process of preventing and healing disease.

CONCLUSION

Voltaire, the eighteenth-century French writer and philosopher, is credited with the statement, "The art of medicine consists in amusing the patient while nature cures the disease." For years, human experience has led people to conclude that laughter is good for their health. This belief is reflected in the well-known *Reader's Digest* feature (borrowed from the ancient proverb) called "Laughter, the Best Medicine." Now we are beginning to empirically demonstrate that laughter is indeed "good medicine." Positive emotions are a wonderful resource of self-generating pharmaceutical benefits within the body. Happiness breeds happiness. Positive emotions and behavior regenerate our cells and invigorate our lives.

The looking forward to and anticipation of positive experiences can potentially facilitate a psychobiology of "hope" for the benefit of mind, body, and spirit.

Norman Cousins, a man with great insight into the relationship between mind and body, stated:

> The best physicians are not just superb diagnosticians but individuals who understand the phenomenal energy (and therefore curative propensity) that flow out of an individual's capacity to retain an optimistic belief and attitude toward problems and human affairs in general. It is a perversion of rationalism to argue that words like "hope" or "faith" or "love" or "grace" [and "laughter"] are without physiological significance. The benevolent emotions are necessary not just because they are pleasant, but because they are regenerative. (1981, pp. 205-224)

An Apache myth relates the following story: The Creator who created human beings, the "two-leggeds," who could do everything. They could talk, walk, run, see, and hear. But The Creator was not satisfied. There was just one more thing he wanted his creature to be able to do, and that was to "laugh." And so men and women laughed and laughed and laughed. It was then that The Creator said, "Now you are fit to live!"

As we embark on the twenty-first century the new tools of molecular biology will provide us with further discoveries in psychoneuroimmunology and the interrelationships between the mind, body, and spirit connections with positive emotions. This will provide us with a greater insight and an appreciation and for the use of complementary/adjunct and integrative (whole person) health and medicine care to serve mankind. After all the medical science may be said and done, "A merry heart doeth good like a medicine."

GUIDED QUESTIONS

1. Discuss general research findings regarding humor and the immune system.
2. State results of the effect anticipation has on mood.
3. State results of the effect anticipation has on the neuroendocrine system.

NOTE

1. Norman Cousins (1979) is known for his book *Anatomy of Illness.* In the mid-1960s he was diagnosed with a degenerative illness and given a few months to live. He fought the illness through a nontraditional approach. He took a high dose of vitamin C and exposed himself to lots of humor.

REFERENCES

Berk, L. S., Felten, D. L., Tan, S. A., Bittman, B., and Westengard, J. (2001). *Modulation of neuroimmune parameters during the eustress or humor associated mirthful laughter.* Loma Linda, CA: Loma Linda University, Center for Neuroimmunology.

Berk, L. S., Felten, D. L., Tan, S. A., and Westengard, J. (2002). Anticipation of a positive humor/laughter eustress event decreases detrimental stress hormones and increases β-endorphin prior to the actual humor experience. Program No. 777.4. *2002 Abstract Viewer/Itinerary Planner.* Washington, DC: Society for Neuroscience.

Berk, L. S., Felten, D. L., and Westengard, J. (2001). The anticipation of a laughter eustress event modulates mood states prior to the actual humor experience [Abstract]. *Society for Neuroscience Abstracts, 27,* 572.

Berk, L. S. and Tan, S. A. (1988a). Humor associated laughter decreases cortisol and increases spontaneous lymphocyte blastogenesis. *Clinical Research, 36,* 435A.

Berk, L. S. and Tan, S. A. (1988b). Humor associated laughter modulates adrenal corticomedullary activity. *The Endocrine Society, Seventieth Annual Meeting, Abstract Supplement,* p. 219.

Berk, L. S. and Tan S. A. (1995). A positive emotion: The eustress of mirthful laughter modulates the immune system lymphokine interferon-gamma. *Psychoneuroimmunology Research Society Annual Meetings, Abstract Supplement*, April 17-20, pp. A.1-A.4.

Berk, L. S., Tan, S. A., and Fry, W. F. (1993). Eustress of humor associated laughter modulates specific immune system components. *Annals of Behavioral Medicine*, 15(Supplement) S111.

Berk, L. S., Tan, S. A., Fry, W. F., Napier, B. J., Lee, J. W., Hubbard, R. W., Lewis, J. E., and Eby, W. C. (1989). Neuroendocrine and stress hormone changes during mirthful laughter. *The American Journal of Medical Science*, 298(6), 390-396.

Berk, L. S., Tan, S. A., Napier, B. J., and Eby, W. C. (1989). Eustress of mirthful laughter modifies natural killer cell activity. *Clinical Research*, 37(1), A115.

Cousins, N. (1979). *Anatomy of an illness as perceived by the patient: Reflections on healing and regeneration*. New York: Norton.

Cousins, N. (1981). *The human option: An autobiographical notebook*. New York: Norton.

Derks, P., Gillikin, L. S., Bartolome-Rull, D. S., and Bogart, E. H. (1997). Laughter and electroencephalographic activity. *Humor*, 10, 285-300.

Rayl, A. J. S. (2000). Humor: A mind-body connection: Will researchers and comedy legends demonstrate laughter's therapeutic qualities? *The Scientist: The News Journal for the Life Scientist*, 14(19), 1-2.

Tan, S. A., Tan, L. G., Berk, L. S., Lukman, S. T., and Lukman, L. F. (1997). Mirthful laughter, an effective adjunct in cardiac rehabilitation. *The Canadian Journal of Cardiology*, 13, 190B, June 1997.

Chapter 3

Spirituality and Coping with Trauma

Brenda Cole
Ethan Benore
Kenneth Pargament

OBJECTIVES

1. To provide an overview of the research literature that will (a) clarify concepts associated with coping, (b) describe the functional qualities of spirituality in the coping process, and (c) outline religious stereotypes and shifts toward a positive view of spirituality.
2. To describe the dual nature of spirituality and associated outcomes.
3. To address the importance of spiritual integration within the framework of spiritual coping and outcomes, and describe the relationship to factors outside and within the larger orienting system.
4. To discuss the practical implications of spiritual coping for health care professionals working in multidisciplinary settings.
5. To discuss interventions for addressing the spiritual needs and concerns of patients.

Correspondence should be addressed to: Brenda Cole, Division of Behavioral Medicine and Oncology, University of Pittsburgh Cancer Institute, Iroquois Building, Suite 405, 3600 Forbes Avenue, Pittsburgh, PA 15213. Phone (412) 624-4871. Fax: (412) 647-1936. Electronic mail may be sent to: bcole@pitt.edu.

INTRODUCTION

Tony had struggled with shyness all her life. Although she was a very spiritual person, had extensively studied several meditative practices, and had a burning desire to teach others what she had learned, her shyness kept her from acting on that goal. When she was diagnosed with thyroid cancer, and warned by her physician that there was a small risk that she could lose her voice as a side effect of treatment, she interpreted her cancer as a spiritual wake-up call: "If I don't use my voice, I'm going to lose it." She coped with her diagnosis by using this interpretation as a motivator; she was determined to take action on her desire to teach. Weeks after completing treatment, which fortunately did not cause any damage to her voice, she led her first healing meditation workshop for a local congregation.

Nancy had postponed other life goals, and had invested most of her adult life in taking care of her family. Her spiritual life was also very important to her and she often volunteered her time to help her church congregation. Just as her last child was preparing to enter college and Nancy was looking forward to finally having "time of her own," she was diagnosed with breast cancer. This event evoked a sense of betrayal: how could God let her get cancer when she had given so much to others, and at a time when she was so eagerly awaiting what she had envisioned as a reward for her devotion and care? Struggling with this issue was painful, but fortunately Nancy's strong commitment to her faith helped her eventually replace her "betrayal" interpretation with one that was congruent with her belief in a loving God: she began to think about how her cancer might have a positive spiritual purpose.

For better or worse, spirituality is often embedded in the process of coping with major life stressors, such as a diagnosis of cancer. Studies have shown that spirituality is among the most common resources people rely upon when they are faced with traumas (Gilbert, 1989; Greil et al., 1989; Pargament et al., 1990). Researchers have begun to identify the rich and varied ways spirituality expresses itself in stressful times. Moreover, they have begun to differentiate healthier from less healthy ways of spiritual coping and apply this knowledge to efforts to treat people dealing with difficult life events, including medical illnesses. In this chapter, we will review this emerging body of literature. We begin with some definitions of our key terms.

DEFINITIONS

Most people do not respond passively to stressful life events, such as a diagnosis of cancer. Even under the most dire circumstances, people typically are proactive, searching for ways to regain or enhance what they hold as important in their lives. That is, they engage in coping, a process we define as "a search for significance in times of stress" (Pargament, 1997, p. 90). It is a process that is active, goal oriented, and value driven. The goals may vary from person to person or event to event. Some people, like Tony, strive for meaning and enhanced spirituality. Other people may strive to regain a sense of control or strengthen intimate connections with loved ones. However, the common aspect that underlies the coping process for each individual is the pursuit of significance, or striving toward goals that are deemed to be most worthy of pursuit. Moreover, because the coping process is value driven, it is not surprising that spirituality is intricately interwoven throughout the process for many people, as is apparent in the previous two stories (see Pargament, 1997 for a review). Spirituality is intimately connected to personal values for most people in our culture. Statistics indicate that up to 95 percent of Americans believe in God, two-thirds generally report having an affiliation with a religious organization, and most people rate religion as "very important" in their lives (Hoge, 1996).

By spirituality, we mean a *search for the sacred*. By "search" we mean efforts to discover, experience, conserve, and/or transform the sacred. By "sacred" we mean those things that are considered to be holy or divine. The "sacred" is most typically associated with theistic figures (e.g., God or Allah), however, nontheistic concepts (life force or energy) may equally represent the sacred. Moreover, mundane objects and experiences may take on sacred character or significance through their association with the divine (Mahoney et al., 1999). For example, for a Buddhist, an area of the home may be made sacred through its designation as a place for spiritual meditation and the presence of spiritually significant pictures or symbols. Although classically, religion has been defined as both an individual and institutional phenomenon, for the purposes of this discussion we will speak of religion in its institutional sense; that is, *organized beliefs and practices based on a social institution and related to the sacred* (see Thoresen, 1999). We will focus largely on spirituality because of its relevance to diverse religious traditions and diverse people coping with adversity.

THE SPIRITUALITY AND COPING CONNECTION

Spirituality can be involved in the coping process in various ways (see Figure 3.1): as a stable resource or burden (Box 1), as an intervention (Box 2), as a coping response (Box 3), or as an outcome (Box 4). One component of stable resources and burdens that is particularly relevant for this chapter is the individual's enduring spiritual orienting system (see Pargament, 1997).

The spiritual orienting system is the worldview that people draw from as a foundation for their lives. It comprises typical behaviors, attitudes, values, patterns of relating to other people, beliefs, and personality. Out of this orienting system of resources and liabilities people select particular ways of spiritual coping with life stressors. Their choice of specific ways of coping has important implications for outcomes and can affect people physically, psychologically, and socially

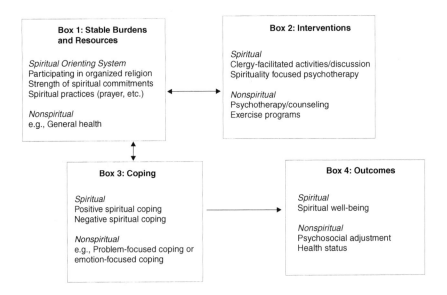

FIGURE 3.1. The Many Aspects of Spirituality Within the Coping Process

(Box 4). But it is also important to recognize that spirituality itself is shaped and reshaped through the coping process. Thus, we can also speak of spiritual outcomes of the coping process.

BEYOND STEREOTYPES

From a psychological standpoint, some people within the field of psychology have viewed religion and spirituality stereotypically as detrimental to psychological health either because it propagates irrational beliefs (Ellis, 1986) or because it functions as a defense mechanism (Freud (1927/1961). Freud was a strong proponent of this latter conceptualization of religion and spirituality. Because he was so influential within the field of psychology, this section will take a critical look at the question of whether spirituality is best understood as a "defense mechanism." Although this argument has been traditionally framed in terms of religion (institutionally and individually), it is just as applicable to the concept of spirituality. Freud argued that spirituality, as we define it, provides its adherents with an irrational belief system that makes life bearable by avoiding the anxiety of problems, denying that "bad things" can happen, and passively (or avoiding altogether) coping with stress and trauma. In line with this theory, it is not difficult to locate individuals who appear to use their spirituality defensively. However, to say that spirituality is *solely* a defense mechanism represents an overstatement, and relies on three stereotypes that have little in the way of empirical support (see Pargament and Park, 1995).

According to one stereotype, spirituality is merely a strategy to avoid anxiety. Certainly, there are examples of people who look to their faith for comfort and solace from their anxiety. However, spirituality has the capacity to increase as well as allay anxiety, as we read in Nancy's story (Pargament, Zinnbauer, et al., 1998). Furthermore, spirituality is a proactive process that provides its followers with a multitude of pathways to pursue goals of ultimate value to them—not simply the avoidance of anxiety. For example, some may use spirituality to search for meaning in life, to enhance their understanding of the world and of themselves. In this vein, one research study found that recent converts to Christianity reported greater purpose in life than nonconverts (Paloutzian, 1981). The converts were not seeking a reduction in distress, but rather an enhanced spiritual life. Spirituality may also help people searching for a sense of unity and intimacy. Through activities within one's church or synagogue, individuals can find a sense of community. Through prayer and rituals, individuals can experience closeness with the Divine. Furthermore, spirituality may assist in the search for self-actualization. Tony had a burning desire to share herself with others as a part of her spiritual journey—to give to others the knowledge she gained through meditative practice.

Research on extrinsic and intrinsic religiousness further challenges the "anxiety reduction" model of spirituality. Allport (1950) described two orientations that individuals may take toward religion. One orientation entails motivation to attain psychological or social goals through religion (extrinsic religiousness), such as reduced distress and a sense of belonging. The second religious orientation involves motivation toward religion as an end in and of itself (intrinsic religiousness). Intrinsically oriented people look to religion to achieve closeness with the Divine or to gain spiritual enlightenment. These orientations to religion are not exclusive—one may be involved in religion for both spiritual and nonspiritual goals. Either way, religious orientations are not, part and parcel, a means of anxiety reduction.

A second stereotype is that spirituality is merely a form of denial. Like many stereotypes, this one may contain a grain of truth. For example, in one study of fundamentalists suffering from terminal cancer, those patients who experienced high levels of support from the church were more likely to deny the illness and risk of mortality than those with less church support (Gibbs and Achterberg-Lawlis, 1978). How does spirituality lead some people to deny what appear to be objective facts? Beliefs in a loving and caring God can provide a powerful mechanism for overlooking a reality (I have cancer) in favor of a perceived spiritual truth (God wouldn't let that happen to me) that affirms one's spiritual commitments. However, to define the function of spirituality solely in terms of denial is an extremely limited view of spiritual life. Spirituality provides a broad orienting system for individuals—a set of core beliefs that help them interpret and cope with various situations (refer to Figure 3.1, Box 1). Out of this orienting system, people can select myriad ways to appraise a negative event. For example, a tragedy can be viewed as one of life's lessons administered by God, or perhaps as a part of God's benevolent plan for humanity. Tony saw her diagnosis of cancer as a wake-up call to pursue a spiritual goal. However, she *reinterpreted* the meaning of her diagnosis rather than denied the diagnosis itself. Positive reframing of this kind has been linked to positive health outcomes, such as self-esteem, psychological adjustment, and personal growth (Jenkins and Pargament, 1988; Park and Cohen, 1993).

A third stereotype is that spirituality is merely a passive, avoidant way of coping with tragedies. The assumption is that when tragedy occurs, the spiritual individual defers problem solving to God and withdraws passively, claiming that "God will take care of me," or that "It is in God's hands now." This stereotypical view is supported by a study by Asser and Swan (1998) who identified 172 children who died from medical illness because their parents refused standard medical care. The overriding rationale of the parents was that they should not interfere with God's divine plan by providing standard medical care to their children.

Deferring to God is one form of coping, but it is not the *only* form of spiritual coping and may not even be the most prevalent form. People often take a more collaborative approach, seeing God as a partner in coping rather than as the sole locus of responsibility or control (Pargament et al., 1988). Moreover, studies have shown how some forms of spiritual coping (e.g., prayer, seeking spiritual support) are negatively related to avoidant forms of coping and positively related to active forms of coping (Pargament and Park, 1995). The argument that spiritual coping is a form of avoidant coping is primarily based on the notion that spirituality discourages personal control. However, studies have shown that some aspects of spirituality (e.g., church attendance, intrinsic religiousness) are related to an increase in personal control. Many people reject the passive deferral of their problems to God. Instead, they view God as working through them, along side of them, or spiritually supporting their individual efforts.

To say that spirituality is merely a way to avoid anxiety, deny reality, or passively cope with life's difficulties oversimplifies the richness and complexity of spiritual life. Spirituality assists individuals in seeking a full range of goals and offers a way to reframe negative events, maintaining a positive outlook during even the darkest of days. In short, spirituality provides people with a variety of pathways for living.

Fortunately, with regard to these historical stereotypes of spirituality and coping in the literature, it appears that the pendulum is beginning to swing the other way—from a reductionist view of spirituality as a defense mechanism, to a multifaceted view of spirituality as providing various pathways to assist individuals striving for the sacred during times of stress. This is not to say that spirituality cannot be detrimental to one's health—for this also may be true. However, to better understand the spiritual lives of individuals encountering a variety of traumas, we need to consider the *variety* of spiritual beliefs and behaviors that contribute to the coping process.

THE TWO FACES OF SPIRITUAL COPING: NEGATIVE AND POSITIVE

The stories of Tony and Nancy suggest that spiritual coping can be either positive or negative in character. Tony's interpretation of her cancer as a spiritual lesson, and the use of that lesson to make important changes in her life presents an image of positive spiritual coping. Moreover, her story suggests that her view of cancer helped her cope with the threat, maintain an optimistic outlook, and minimize the impact of her cancer on her future psychological, and thus potentially, her physical health. Nancy's story, on the other hand, included struggling spiritually in her coping. The result of this struggle, at least initially, seemed to be additional distress. Her way of making sense out of cancer (i.e., seeing it as a betrayal by God) may have temporarily exacerbated not only her psychological distress, but also her physical symptomatology.

Consistent with these two stories, research on spiritual coping has identified two different patterns of spiritual coping: positive and negative (Pargament, Smith, et al., 1998). Notably, both of these forms of coping are based on theistic concepts of the sacred. Positive spiritual coping involves strategies that reflect a benevolent and supportive image of God and the spiritual community. These strategies include spiritual forgiveness, seeking spiritual support, collaborative coping, spiritual connection, and benevolent spiritual reappraisals. *Spiritual forgiveness* involves seeking forgiveness from God as well as seeking God's help in letting go of anger toward others. This can be sought in various ways, such as discussion with clergy, prayer or meditation, or rituals. *Seeking spiritual support* involves seeking love and care from God. *Collaborative coping* refers to thinking of God as an active partner who is working with the person to put his or her coping plans into action. *Spiritual connection* refers to seeking a stronger connection with God. This can be done through religious services, prayer or meditation, or reading spiritual material. *Benevolent reappraisals* involve positive interpretations of the event as holding a spiritual lesson or benefit.

Negative spiritual coping refers to strategies that reflect spiritual isolation and conflict. They include spiritual discontent, punishing God reappraisals, interpersonal spiritual discontent, demonic reappraisals, and reappraisals of God's power. *Spiritual discontent* refers to questioning God's love or interpreting the event as abandonment from God. This was the interpretation used by Nancy to make sense of her breast cancer diagnosis. *Interpersonal spiritual discontent* refers to conflicts with a religious community or feelings of spiritual abandonment. *Demonic reappraisals* involve interpreting the event as the work of the devil. *Punishing God reappraisals* involve interpreting the event as a punishment from God for one's sins or lack of spiritual devotion. *Reappraisals of God's power* involve considering that God may not be all powerful. Rather than attributing the event to God's punishment, God can be reappraised as unable to prevent terrible events from occurring.

These positive and negative approaches to spiritual coping have different implications for how well people recover from the event. People who use positive spiritual coping when they are confronted with a stressful life event report more positive outcomes, including stress-related growth, both spiritual and secular. These findings have emerged in studies of people experiencing a variety of stressful life events, including the devastating bombing of the Murrah Federal Building in Oklahoma City in 1995 or hospitalization for medical problems (Pargament, Smith, et al., 1998). For example, the person who turns to God for comfort and support is more likely to say, "The event taught me to be myself more rather than trying to live up to other people's expectations," "I learned to be more confident," "I learned how to reach out and help others," or "I grew spiritually."

People using negative spiritual coping do not fare nearly as well. They voice more emotional distress. Of even more concern is some evidence suggesting that negative spiritual coping may lead to poorer health outcomes. People using negative spiritual coping to cope with a variety of stressful life events (e.g., hospitalization) report poorer physical health and higher levels of psychosomatic symptoms (Koenig,

Pargament, and Nielsen, 1998; Pargament, Smith, et al., 1998). For example, in work with cancer patients, negative spiritual coping strategies were linked to greater depression and anxiety, and more frequent pain (Cole et al., 1998).

Of course, in cross-sectional research, we cannot tell whether the negative spiritual coping is causing people to be more distressed and report more pain, or the pain and distress are leading to more negative spiritual coping. Because they are suffering, people may be more likely to interpret their situations in terms of being abandoned or punished by God. However, two separate longitudinal studies suggest spiritual coping is causally linked to poorer outcomes. In one study, medical rehabilitation patients who reported more use of negative spiritual coping at the time of their admission to a rehabilitation center, had more difficulty recovering physical functioning after four months (Fitchett et al., 1999). In another study, Pargament and several other colleagues assessed spiritual coping used by hospitalized elderly patients. They found that the more negative spiritual coping the patients were using during the initial hospitalization, the greater the risk of mortality during the next two years (Pargament et al., 2001).

Although it is tempting to conclude that negative spiritual coping is bad for one's health and positive spiritual coping is good, this would be too simplistic for several reasons. First, the study of spiritual coping using scientifically rigorous methods is a relatively new undertaking in psychology and health. Certainly additional studies are needed before coming to such definitive conclusions. Second, the impact of negative spiritual coping may vary depending on when it occurs during the coping process and how long it lasts. Initial feelings of betrayal by God, such as those experienced by Nancy, may not have long-lasting negative consequences if that sense of betrayal is short lived and a more benign interpretation is constructed. In this vein, researchers have found that negative spiritual coping is linked not only to physical and emotional distress, but also to stress-related growth. Thus, it may be more accurate to consider negative spiritual coping as a "red flag" that should be explored as a potentially problematic response to stressors (Pargament, Zinnbauer, et al., 1998). Finally, spiritual coping is just one aspect of the coping process (refer back to Figure 3.1, Box 1 and 3). The effects of spiritual coping are intertwined with other elements. A more complete evaluation of the value of spiritual coping also requires an assessment of the degree to which spiritual coping is integrated in the larger coping process. The next section will explore this topic.

ASSESSING SPIRITUAL INTEGRATION

Spiritual coping is often helpful in reducing distress and enhancing adjustment to tragic events, but sometimes spiritual coping goes awry. Pargament (1997) provides a conceptual framework to answer the question: How does spiritual coping go wrong? This framework delineates how spiritual coping can become ineffective, and even detrimental, when the individual is unable to *integrate* the various aspects of his or her spiritual life. "Spiritual disintegration" can occur both within the coping process (Figure 3.1, Box 3) and within the broader spiritual orienting system (Figure 3.1, Box 1). We will explore these two areas in turn. First, we describe three problems associated with spiritual disintegration within the coping process—the "wrong direction," the "wrong road," and "against the stream." We then describe how disintegration in the larger spiritual orienting system influences the coping process.

Disintegration in the Coping Process

The first problem in spiritual coping is called the "wrong direction." This occurs when the destinations, goals, or purposes in one's life are not well integrated. If one's goals in life are not in harmony with one another, problems can arise. For example, Goodman et al. (1991) observed that elderly Jewish mothers had greater difficulty adjusting to the death of their adult children than non-Jewish mothers. Further study revealed that the Jewish mothers were focused on the well-being of their children to the exclusion of other goals and values. The loss of their children symbolized the loss of their central purpose in life, and they had little else in their lives to balance the effects of this trauma. Life can also become unbalanced when a spiritual goal becomes the individual's exclusive focus of attention.

This one-sided view of spirituality can take many forms. Pargament (1997) wrote, "Any end, even the most virtuous, can become problematic when pursued to the exclusion of other values" (p. 320).

To restate, when individuals place all their energy in the pursuit of one rigid spiritual goal, other aspects of life are likely to suffer. It is important to emphasize that we are not speaking against religious fervor, but pointing out the potential for problems when other values in life are excluded in the pursuit of rigid spiritual ones.

Another form of "wrong directions" in spiritual coping involves religious deception. Spiritual goals may appear noble at the surface level, but it is possible that deeper motives drive individual behaviors. Many are skeptical of televangelists asking for monetary donations. Do they want to save souls or just make a quick buck? But deception does not need to occur on a grand scheme. Some people may rely on "spiritual principles" to support otherwise intolerable behavior, such as oppression, prejudice, and abuse of others, both within and outside of their spiritual system. During the Civil War, for example, scriptural citations were commonly used to justify slavery. Some individuals may be victims of their own self-deception—denying their true motives for spiritual behavior.

A second problem in spiritual coping has been called the "wrong road" (Pargament, 1997). People taking the wrong road may have well-integrated values and direction in life, but the methods they take to reach their goals are not integrated with other behaviors. For example, an individual could endorse a spiritual appraisal for events and exclude other equally valid explanations, with resulting negative outcomes. For example, believing an illness is a punishment from God, and excluding other potential explanations such as a genetic predisposition, limits coping options and may compromise psychological, spiritual, and potentially, physical well-being.

Taking the "wrong road" is also evident when perceptions of personal control do not match the actual level of control available to the individual in the situation. On one hand, individuals may view themselves as having much less control over the situation than is actually the case. When individuals perceive they have too little control over a stressor, they may rely exclusively on spiritual coping strategies, and defer all effort to control the situation to God or other spiritual powers. As Asser and Swan (1998) reported, families who interpreted physical illness as curable only through divine interventions tended to neglect the resources of modern medicine and, as a result, suffered many preventable deaths. On the other hand, it is also possible to perceive too much control over some events, specifically when the event is uncontrollable. A patient suffering terminal illness may fight desperately and for many months for additional medical treatments to no avail. This futile struggle to control illness is likely to cause greater anxiety, anger, and sadness, as well as distract from pursuing other meaningful aspects of life, such as family relationships. Thus, both overcontrol and undercontrol can result in "wrong roads" of coping. The better way is nicely articulated in the Serenity Prayer: "God grant me the serenity to accept the things I cannot change, courage to change the things I can, and wisdom to know the difference."

One additional example of taking the "wrong road" includes extreme modes of spiritual coping. When a spiritual goal is pursued too intensely, other aspects of life may be devalued. For example, a person may stop at nothing to protect the sanctity of unborn life, even if it means murdering individuals at an abortion clinic. However, extremism can also be present in apathy. Spiritual goals may *not* be pursued, despite the significance they hold for an individual. For example, a family may not speak out for peace and community in their neighborhood, for fear of becoming a target of violent delinquent activity. In summary then, the wrong road in spiritual coping can involve a one-sided interpretation of the stressful event, a one-sided approach to coping (e.g., attempting to exert too much personal control), or an extremist position.

A final problem in spiritual coping is best described as coping "against the stream" (Pargament, 1997). In this case, the lack of integration does not lie within an individual, but between an individual and his or her religious system. For example, a member of a pro-life religious community (e.g., Roman Catholicism) may have an abortion and, subsequently, feel more guilty, depressed, and isolated from her community than one who does not belong to that spiritual group (see Osofsky and Osofsky, 1972; Payne et al., 1976). Going "against the stream" can have even stronger implications for minority religions that suffer intolerance within the larger social system. For example, if Tony practiced Hinduism in a predominantly Christian community, pursuing her spiritual goal of teaching might be more difficult. The costs of going against the stream may be high. However, a lack of spiritual fit may also entail benefits such as greater perceived control and self-efficacy. Moreover, not fitting within the religious system may create an impetus for change within the social system and promote more adaptive behaviors within the spiritual community as a whole.

These problems encountered in spiritual coping—"wrong direction," "wrong road," and "against the stream"—are influenced by the larger orienting system of the individual. We now turn to discuss disintegration within that system.

Disintegration Within the Orienting System

The orienting system comprises the spiritual aspect of the stable burdens and resources that individuals bring to the coping process (see Figure 3.1, Box 1). It provides the foundation of coping and includes core beliefs and values that guide how people perceive and interact with the world. Coping involves organizing and using these resources to overcome stressful life experiences (Pargament, 1997). If the orienting system is strong, well developed, and well integrated, coping is more adaptive. However, when the system is lacking these qualities, coping may become ineffective or even detrimental. Four forms of spiritual disintegration within the orienting system are described as follows.

First, spirituality may become undifferentiated or one-sided. This involves pursuing one narrow aspect of one's faith, or ignoring the full spectrum of one's faith. An individual with undifferentiated spirituality cannot tell "the forest from the trees" when using spirituality to cope with life stress. Therefore, the individual is unable to produce a variety of coping responses. For example, an individual may view spirituality as complete submission to God's will, forfeiting any sense of personal control. Baider and De-Nour (1987) described several Arab Muslims with breast cancer who believed their cancer was God's will and did nothing to assist in timely diagnosis and treatment of the cancer. Also, undifferentiated spirituality may involve ignoring challenging or negative aspects of spiritual life. Many people will endorse positive statements about their faith and avoid difficult spiritual questions or conflicts (Pargament, 1997). Therefore, positive change to correct or improve their spiritual orienting system is unlikely to occur. Furthermore, undifferentiated spirituality may take a fatalistic point of view. Individuals may attend to the negative side of spiritual life (e.g., punishment, hell), but ignore aspects of spiritual redemption. As an example, Watson, Morris, and Hood (1988) demonstrated that spiritual guilt was related to negative life outcomes; however, those who also believed in grace reported better outcomes.

A second form of spiritual disintegration is fragmented spirituality. Fragmentation occurs when there is a gap between what one says, does, and believes. These fragmented pieces of one's spirituality may be unable to provide stable support in times of stress. For example, individuals may separate their spirituality from many other aspects of daily life. Some professed Christians attend church only on Christmas and Easter and seldom apply their faith to life circumstances. Also, people may feel a sense of peace and communion within the church walls only to curse at fellow churchgoers when trying to exit the crowded church parking lot. In addition, spiritual beliefs may be disconnected from spiritual practices. Individuals who feel that their faith rituals are hollow activities may have difficulty when attempting to rely on their faith in times of stress. Spirituality as practiced may be divorced from the sacred in one's life and, as a result, spiritual coping may feel hollow and pointless. Of course, anyone's spirituality is likely to have *some* inconsistencies or fragmentation. When fragmentation becomes too great the potential for problems in coping occurs.

Third, spirituality may be inflexible. Spiritual flexibility allows the individual to adapt to new stressful situations with new modes of coping. Flexible spirituality does not mean "soft" or weak ways of relating to the sacred. Rather, flexibility allows an individual to utilize different perspectives to interpret the stressful event and different strategies to cope with it. An example of inflexible spirituality is extreme spiritual fundamentalism that may support prejudice and intolerance in some believers, as illustrated by a fundamentalist who views AIDS as "God's punishment" for homosexual behaviors. Nancy's story also portrays an initially inflexible religious interpretation of her diagnosis. To protect inflexible spiritual standards, many will lash out in anger at threats to their faith, which can compound, rather than diminish, their problems.

Finally, an individual may have an insecure spiritual attachment. For individuals who have a theistic orientation, God acts as a significant attachment figure (Kirkpatrick and Shaver, 1992). Like parental attachment, a secure spiritual attachment may allow individuals to feel supported by God and evoke supportive and collaborative strategies to cope with stressful events. On the other hand, people may also develop an insecure attachment. Here, they may feel alienated from the sacred and distrustful that God will be there for them through tough times (see Kirkpatrick and Shaver, 1992). This alienation may extend to estrangement from the spiritual community. In this situation, spirituality may be unable to provide a stable resource that can buffer the individual against the stress. Here, the individual is likely to feel heightened anxiety, ambivalence toward spiritual resources, or may use spiritual coping methods in a less effective and potentially harmful manner.

In summary, although spiritual coping can benefit individuals, disintegration can lead to problems in the coping process in two ways that may, in turn, lead to less favorable outcomes. First, disintegration can be evident in the "flow of coping"; specifically, in the goals sought ("wrong direction"), the methods used ("wrong road"), or the individual's fit within the larger system ("against the stream"). Second, disintegration can be evident within the spiritual orienting system that provides the foundation for coping. A lack of integration is evident in this system when it becomes one-sided or fragmented, adopts an inflexible view of spirituality, or is marked by insecure spiritual attachments. Disintegration within the orienting system is likely to undermine the coping process, increasing the difficulty that people experience when confronted by trauma and leading to poorer outcomes (Box 4). Thus, a relevant goal within physical and mental health care settings is to identify individuals who are struggling with these issues and to intervene in a helpful manner in order to promote positive spiritual coping and better adjustment. This topic will be addressed in the next section.

CLINICAL IMPLICATIONS

As noted, most people rely on spiritual coping when facing stressful life events. Moreover, most people perceive spiritual coping to be helpful and research suggests that, for the majority of people, spiritual coping is well integrated in the overall coping process. However, for a minority of people, with estimates around 25 percent, spiritual problems are evident and expressed as spiritual conflicts or strain (Fitchett et al., 1999). An important clinical agenda is to identify these individuals and intervene in an ethical and helpful manner. This section will discuss ways to accomplish these two goals.

Identifying the presence of spiritual problems is complicated by tight disciplinary boundaries that place spiritual issues and concerns solely within the purview of pastoral care. Multidisciplinary health care teams that operate within hospital settings are helping to redefine these boundaries. Physicians, nurses, psychologists, clergy, and ethicists are often included on these teams, and they work together to provide holistic care that responds to the diverse psychological, physical, and spiritual needs of the patient. Each team member brings unique expertise to the process and takes on a more active, or less active and more consultative role depending on the needs of the patient. Professional boundaries need to be more fluid for the team to operate effectively. For example, the nurse who is most familiar to the patient may be the best person to initiate a psychological intervention in consultation with the team psychologist to decrease anticipatory anxiety and increase patient comfort prior to a difficult medical procedure. At other times, the distress may be too great and better managed directly by the team psychologist. Likewise, spiritual issues may be best addressed by various members of the medical team depending on the patient. A patient who is well-grounded in a particular faith may welcome a visit from pastoral care and experience it as comforting. However, a patient who has lingering guilt or anger over previous wounds attributed to a religious organization may find such a visit intrusive and distressing. Spiritual issues may contribute to this patient's distress, especially if the illness is life threatening or severely debilitating. However, a physician or nurse may be the best person to initiate a discussion of these issues, and if an intervention seems warranted and the patient agrees, a psychologist may be in a better position to assist the patient in resolving his or her spiritual distress. In this scenario, clergy may best function in a consultative role.

This multidisciplinary model with semipermeable boundaries guided the development of this section of the chapter. It is a model that applies not only to inpatient health care settings, but to outpatient settings, and community settings as well. Most people in the United States participate in an interconnected system of mental, physical, and spiritual care professionals. The system may be well integrated (as in the hospital setting) or less integrated (when little or no exchange occurs between the various providers). Care is optimized when professionals within various disciplines assess needs across disciplines, address those needs to the extent possible within their own discipline (considering professional roles, the patient's unique characteristics, and needs), and consult with or refer to other professionals as warranted by the patient's preferences and needs.

To do this ethically and sensitively, several precautions need to be taken. First and foremost, ethical spiritual care requires respecting and honoring the spiritual or religious beliefs and commitments of the patient. Proselytizing is exploitative, coercive (especially with highly vulnerable patients), and unacceptable. It is important to recognize your own personal biases, whether you are a devout Roman Catholic or atheist, and take steps to ensure that they are not conveyed to the patient. This will require monitoring your intonation and body language when asking about spiritual needs and concerns to convey an attitude of acceptance and support. If a professional cannot do this, clearly he or she should not address spiritual issues. Second, develop expertise in integrating spirituality in your work. If you are going to explore spiritual issues with a patient or client it is important to obtain training and or supervision to ensure that you are integrating spiritual issues in a way that is ethical and congruent with the patient's needs. The degree of training needed will vary depending on the extent to which spiritual dimensions are addressed in your work. Minimal training might suffice for a physician or nurse to assess spiritual needs in order to determine the need for a referral. However, more extensive training would be necessary to administer a spiritual intervention. Spiritual interventions are most appropriate when delivered within pastoral care, psychotherapy, or identified spiritual growth/ support groups. Of course, these interventions should be initiated only after informed consent has been obtained. Third, keep in mind that patients may not need answers related to their spiritual conflicts or concerns as much as a sensitive, encouraging, listening ear. Two recent studies have found positive benefits when physicians simply asked medically ill patients about spiritual issues (Rhodes and Kristeller, 2000; Norum, Risberg, and Solberg, 2000). As an example of the benefits, Rhodes and Kristeller found that cancer patients were more satisfied with their medical care and communication with their oncologists when the doctor spent a few minutes with them asking them about spiritual or religious concerns. These patients, compared to those who were not asked about spiritual issues, showed greater decreases in depression and more improved quality of life.

The first step in addressing spiritual concerns is to assess their relevancy for patients. This can be done very simply and unintrusively as part of an overall assessment by asking three very brief questions.

1. *Is spirituality or religion important to you?* If they answer "no," discontinue this line of questioning, otherwise continue. In our experience, the answer to this question will help you pinpoint whether patients see themselves as more spiritual or more religious. Use the term most relevant to the patients as you continue.
2. *Are there ways that your spirituality (religion) has been helpful to you as you have coped with your illness (trauma)?*
3. *Do you have any spiritual questions or challenges that are causing you some concern?*

In addition, if spiritual questions or challenges are acknowledged, consider the administration of a measure of spiritual well-being developed specifically for people who have experienced a stressful life event, such as the Spiritual Affect Scale (Cole and Baum, 2002). This scale is appropriate for people who have a relational concept of the sacred (God, higher power, Allah, life force, etc.) and assesses the affective qualities of that relationship (i.e., the extent to which the person feels positive affect such as feeling comforted or feels negative affect such as feeling punished). Endorsement of any of the negative affect items (feeling angry, hurt, punished, abandoned, shameful, or distant) signals the presence of spiritual distress and suggests the need to explore this further with the patient and discuss available resources to resolve this distress. The Brief RCOPE, a measure of negative and positive spiritual coping, could also be administered to identify the use of problematic spiritual coping strategies (Pargament, Smith, et al., 1998). Beyond initial assessments, and as part of ongoing medical or mental health care, it is important for practitioners to continue to listen for signs of spiritual distress. Patients reluctant to discuss spiritual issues may only reveal problematic spiritual issues in subtle ways through the course of treatment. Moreover, as circumstances change, spiritual issues may become more relevant.

Spiritually focused interventions may be helpful for people coping with traumatic events. Interventions that integrate spiritual themes and resources are culturally sensitive to the preferences and needs of spiritually oriented people. A small survey of thirty-six people with cardiac syncope found that most (78 percent) preferred psychotherapy programs that included a spiritual focus (Cole, Pargament, and Brownstein, 2000). More data are needed before firm conclusions can be made; however, our clinical experience and that of others supports this observation: Spiritual people prefer to have spirituality integrated in their care. These types of programs may be beneficial as preventative measures delivered to people regardless of the presence of spiritual or psychological distress. But even more important, when spiritual distress is present, integrating spiritual concerns and exploring spiritual resolutions are especially relevant and may be essential to improving not only spiritual, but also physical and psychological well-being.

Spiritually focused interventions can take many forms and only a few of the most frequently used forms will be reviewed here. Less structured approaches involve individual interventions delivered by clergy or mental health professions. Historically, spiritual interventions have been implemented through private counseling with a member of the clergy or through traditional religious rituals and practices. These types of interventions are likely to be most helpful for people who are already grounded in and committed to a particular religious orientation. A second alternative involves spiritually integrative psychotherapy with a mental health professional. The therapist can assist the individual in identifying problems with integration (e.g., wrong direction or wrong road circumstances), exploring deficiencies in their spiritual orienting system (e.g., spiritual inflexibility or too great a discrepancy between spiritual beliefs and behaviors), adopting more positive rather than negative spiritual coping strategies (e.g., transforming an image of a punishing God to an image of a loving and supporting God), and resolving negative affect related to the sacred (e.g., replacing feelings of anger and hurt with feelings of being blessed and comforted).

Interventions using a more structured format have also been reported in the literature. Clergy and mental health professionals have historically used meditation to enhance both spiritual and psychological well-being. It most often involves focusing the attention on an image, a physical sensation such as breathing, a mantra (i.e., repeated sound or word), or object. Studies have found that meditation is helpful in reducing both psychological and physical stress (see Harris et al., 1999). Moreover, specific to coping with trauma, meditation has helped alleviate emotional distress related to cancer and physical stress symptoms (Speca et al., 2000). Current studies have not shown if the stress reductive aspect of meditation or the associated spiritual aspects alleviate stress. However, meditation is likely to be particularly helpful in enhancing spiritual well-being if the language and imagery employed is spiritual in nature and congruent with the patient's spiritual struggle experience. For example, focusing on being surrounded by God's loving presence may be more helpful than focusing on the breath when the patient is struggling with spiritual alienation.

Forgiveness interventions may also play a role in the recovery from trauma. Recently, psychologists have designed and tested structured forgiveness interventions from a secular point of view. However, the practice of forgiveness has a long history within most religious traditions and most spiritual people are likely to associate forgiveness interventions with their spiritual lives. Forgiveness is a relevant goal for many trauma situations in which a person has been the victim of perceived abandonment, negligence, or assault. Events such as infidelity, divorce, sexual assault, parental abandonment or abuse, discrimination, and acts of war can leave the victim feeling angry, resentful, revengeful, and powerless. These lingering emotions may take their toll on physical, psychological, and spiritual well-being. Forgiveness interventions help the victim to move from these powerful negative emotional states to a sense of compassion, release, healing, and restored hope. This is a new and relatively unexplored area, but pilot research is beginning to suggest that structured forgiveness interventions can have a positive impact by decreasing depression and anxiety and increasing self-esteem, hope, and a positive attitude toward the offender (Enright and Fitzgibbons, 2000).

Although forgiveness intervention models vary somewhat across researchers, interventions typically strive to decrease the negative affect held toward a perpetrator of a wrong (e.g., anger and resentment). Some interventions also strive to increase beneficence, i.e., the extent to which positive feelings and desires are extended toward the wrongdoer. Various components are included in the interventions to reach these goals. Most often, the interventions begin by helping the participant to consider the consequences of *not* forgiving and to consider making a commitment to forgive the offender. If forgiveness is chosen as a personal goal, the process of forgiveness begins. This process most often includes strategies to increase empathy and compassion toward the perpetrator of the wrong. It might include seeing the perpetrator from a broader perspective, for example, considering what life was and is like for him or her and considering that he or she has both good and bad qualities. Some interventions also focus on identifying and replacing negative thoughts toward the perpetrator or foster an awareness that all people have inherent unconditional worth, including the perpetrator. Spiritual aspects can be brought into the process by: reflecting on religious scriptures and or spiritual practices promoting forgiveness, considering God's love for every person, seeing oneself as a loving member of a spiritual family that includes the perpetrator, drawing on a sense of spiritual support in doing the difficult work of forgiveness, and by reflecting on the spiritual meaning of both the wrong and the act of forgiveness (Enright and Fitzgibbons, 2000; Rye and Pargament, 2002).

As a last example of spiritual interventions, several researchers have developed structured cognitive-behavioral therapy programs that integrate psychotherapy and spirituality. Cognitive-behavioral therapy (CBT) refers to a therapy orientation that focuses on changing thoughts, images, and behaviors in ways that lead to a better psychological adjustment. Propst and her colleagues (Propst, 1980; Propst et al., 1992) developed a program for people with depression that presented psychotherapy techniques within a spiritual and religious framework. The therapeutic elements included cognitive-behavioral therapy strategies that have an established history of being helpful in alleviating depression. In one study (Propst, 1980), the techniques involved teaching people how certain thoughts and images (e.g., especially negative thoughts and images about oneself, the world, or the future) lead to depressive feelings. Spirituality was integrated in the intervention by having the participants substitute the negative thoughts/images with corrective thoughts/images that involved spiritual content. For example, using this model, a woman who visualized herself as incompetent in social situations and likely to be rejected might be coached to imagine a social situation including the related negative thoughts about incompetence and rejection, and then transform the image to a more supportive spiritual image: imagining Jesus present with her as she interacted with her friends, supporting her by reminding her that she is a child of God, with unique positive qualities, much loved, and worthy of positive regard from others. Propst and colleagues tested this type of intervention in two studies; in both, the intervention was effective in reducing depression, with some evidence suggesting that it might be more helpful than CBT interventions that do not include the spiritual components (Propst, 1980; Propst et al., 1992).

Cole and colleagues (Cole, Pargament, and Brownstein, 2000; Cole et al., 1998) tested a similar type of intervention for groups of people coping with health problems: cancer and cardiac syncope. The intervention involved using a CBT format to help participants resolve existential issues related to being diagnosed with a serious health problem. These issues included: the loss of control, the need to find meaning, the impact on relationships, and the impact on identity. CBT elements likely to be helpful in resolving these issues were introduced to the participants through weekly two-hour sessions that lasted for about a two-month period. Spirituality was integrated in the program by having participants consider spiritual issues related to each of the themes and to draw on spiritual resources to work toward a satisfactory resolution of these themes. The results suggested that the spiritual intervention buffered the effects of the illness for cancer patients, holding their depression at a constant level, while it escalated for the control group. However, when the intervention was provided to cardiac syncope patients, who tended to suffer from anxiety rather than depression, a different set of results emerged. The spiritual intervention did not have any effects on anxiety or depression; in contrast, a nonspiritual CBT version of the intervention did decrease anxiety. The comparison of these results suggests that the helpfulness of this type of spiritual intervention will likely depend on the type of stressor people are facing.

During the intervention, one session focused on issues related to control. In this session, participants were asked to list those concerns that they felt were under their control or under God's control (a strategy borrowed from Baugh, 1988). To enhance active problem solving the participants first considered the concerns under their control and discussed with the group ways to manage those concerns in a helpful way. They then closed their eyes, imagined taking the proactive steps they had discussed with the group as a way of practicing their plan, and envisioned God beside them as their problem-solving partner, offering guidance and support. Mike, a participant with lung cancer, worked on his concern about the lack of communication between himself and his wife about his cancer. He envisioned having a helpful talk with her, sharing his concerns and feelings. The next week Mike reported back to the group that he had gone home, talked to his wife, and felt less alone.

Next, the participants focused on the issues not under their control and discussed the helpfulness of surrendering or giving up these concerns to God. They then took part in a guided imagery exercise in which they envisioned God present with them, asked God what they needed to surrender and then, if they were ready, envisioned placing this concern in God's hands. Marty, a woman with breast cancer who had been having uncontrollable nausea and vomiting related to her chemotherapy, completed the guided imagery. For this woman "taking charge" had been her typical way of coping most of her life, and, although it often meant that she neglected her emotional life, it was in many respects a helpful strategy for her. As she started the surrender exercise she anticipated that God would tell her to let go of "taking control." She decided, at the group leader's suggestion, to put aside her expectation and see what came up for her. To Marty's astonishment, when she posed the question to God, "What do I most need to surrender?" she saw written on the wall in bold red and black letters, the word "FEAR." Tears streamed down her face as she told the group about her image, and for the first time she admitted to herself and to them that she was absolutely terrified of the chemotherapy and of how ill it was making her. Throughout the rest of the sessions she continued to share more of her emotional reactions with the group, and during the last session, reported for the first time that she had gained a sense of peace: "Somehow, I know now that no matter what happens, nausea or no nausea, I have a spiritual peace that will always be with me." Perhaps coincidentally, or perhaps relatedly, her nausea symptoms decreased in intensity throughout the rest of her chemotherapy.

CONCLUSION

Metaphorically, spirituality is painted into the "picture of coping" in many varied images, brushed from a multicolored palate and splashed with each individual's own unique style. People encounter coping situations against the backdrop of their stable burdens and resources as depicted in Figure 3.1. These resources and burdens compose the landscape from which the coping picture emerges. As part of this armament, the spiritual orienting system provides a framework that colors how people will approach the task of coping with a stressful life event. This system may negatively influence the coping process if it is too one sided, too inflexible, too fragmented, or if the person's relationship with the sacred (e.g., God) is marked by insecurity. From out of this landscape, the coping strategies and themes comprise the action and movement that give the coping process life and meaning. As we have seen, they may involve problematic themes reflective of taking the wrong road, the wrong direction, or going against the grain. If we look closely at the details expressed in the coping portrait, we can identify coping strategies that may be either negative or positive in tone, marked by thoughts of punishment or abandonment, or visions of a higher purpose and a comforting God, respectively. Finally, as we step back and take in the entire panoramic view of the coping process we may get a sense of how all these aspects of the coping process interact to lead to outcomes. Just as all the colors and hues interact to create the mood in a landscape, all these spiritual dimensions of the coping process interact and create the coping outcome. For some people, like Tony, that outcome is optimistic and hopeful. For others, the picture is far more bleak. Regardless of the outcome, to fully understand how spirituality is a part of the coping picture requires going beyond the limited conceptualization of spirituality as a defense mechanism, and looking more carefully at the rich and intricate ways that one's spiritual life is alive throughout the process of coping. Finally, health professionals are beginning to learn how they too can contribute to the picture of spiritual coping in ways that may enhance the color and texture of people's lives.

GUIDED QUESTIONS

1. Name three stereotypical ways people often view spiritual coping.
2. Explain differences between positive and negative spiritual coping.
3. Describe four forms of spiritual disintegration within the orienting system.
4. What is CBT? Offer explanation of its methodology.

REFERENCES

Allport, G. W. (1950). *The individual and his religion: A psychological interpretation.* New York: Macmillan.

Asser, S. M. and Swan, R. (1998). Child fatalities from religion-motivated medical neglect. *Pediatrics,* 101, 625-629.

Baider, L. and De-Nour, A. K. (1987). The meaning of a disease: An exploratory study of Moslem Arab women after a mastectomy. *Journal of Psychosocial Oncology,* 4, 1-13.

Baugh, J. (1988). Gaining control by giving up control: Strategies for coping with powerlessness. In W. L. Miller and J. E. Martin (Eds.), *Behavior therapy and religion: Integrating spiritual and behavioral approaches to change* (pp. 125-138). Newbury Park, CA: Sage Publications.

Cole, B. and Baum, A. (2002). *The spiritual affect scale: A measure of the affective quality of spiritual relationships.* Manuscript submitted for publication, University of Pittsburgh.

Cole, B., Pargament, K., and Brownstein, S. (2000). A spiritually integrative psychotherapeutic intervention for persons with cardiac syncopy. Paper presented at the annual meeting of the American Psychological Association, Washington, DC, August 5.

Cole, B., Pargament, K., Rothfuss, T., and Smith, C. (1998). The integration of spirituality in psychotherapy for people diagnosed with cancer. Paper presented at the annual meeting of the American Psychological Association, San Francisco, California, August 14.

Ellis, A. (1986). *The case against religion: A psychotherapist's view and the case against religiosity.* Austin: American Atheist Press.

Enright, R. and Fitzgibbons, R. (2000). *Helping clients forgive: An empirical guide for resolving anger and restoring hope.* Washington, DC: American Psychological Association.

Fitchett, G., Rybarczyk, B., DeMarco, G., and Nicholas, J. (1999). The role of religion in medical rehabilitation outcomes: A longitudinal study. *Rehabilitation Psychology,* 44(4), 333-353.

Freud, S. (1927/1961). *The future of an illusion.* New York: Norton.

Gibbs, H. W. and Achterberg-Lawlis, J. (1978). Spiritual values and death anxiety: Implications for counseling with terminal cancer patients. *Journal of Counseling Psychology,* 25, 563-569.

Gilbert, K. (1989). Religion as a resource for bereaved parents as they cope with the death of their child. Paper presented at the meeting of the National Council on Family Relations, New Orleans, Louisiana, November.

Goodman, M., Rubinstein, R. L., Alexander, B. B., and Luborsky, M. (1991). Cultural differences among elderly women in coping with the death of an adult child. *Journal of Gerontology: Social Sciences,* 6, S321-329.

Greil, A., Porter, K., Leitko, T., and Riscilli, C. (1989). Why me? Theodicies of infertile women and men. *Sociology of Health and Illness,* 11, 213-229.

Harris, A., Thoresen, C., McCullough, M., and Larson, D. (1999). Spiritually and religiously oriented health interventions. *Journal of Health Psychology,* 4(3), 413-433.

Hoge, D. (1996). Religion in America: The demographics of belief and affiliation. In E. Shafranske (Ed.), *Religion and the clinical practice of clinical psychology* (pp. 21-41). Washington, DC: American Psychological Association.

Jenkins, R. and Pargament, K. I. (1988). The relationship between cognitive appraisals and psychological adjustment in cancer patients. *Social Science and Medicine,* 26, 625-633.

Kirkpatrick, L. A. and Shaver, P. R. (1992). An attachment-theoretical approach to romantic love and religious belief. *Personality and Social Psychology Bulletin,* 18, 266-275.

Koenig, H., Pargament, K., and Nielsen, J. (1998). Religious coping and health status in medically ill hospitalized older adults. *The Journal of Nervous and Mental Disorders,* 186(9), 513-521.

Mahoney, A. M., Pargament, K. I., Jewell, T., Swank, A. B., Scott, E., Emery, E., and Rye, M. (1999). Marriage and the spiritual realm: The role of proximal and distal religious constructs in marital functioning. *Journal of Family Psychology,* 13, 321-338.

Norum, J., Risberg, T., and Solberg, E. (2000). Faith among patients with advanced cancer. A pilot study on patients offered "no more than" palliation. *Support Care Cancer,* 8, 110-114.

Osofsky, J. D. and Osofsky, H. J. (1972). The psychological reaction of parents to legalized abortion. *American Journal of Orthopsychiatry,* 42, 48-60.

Paloutzian, R. F. (1981). Purpose in life and value changes following conversion. *Journal of Personality and Social Psychology,* 41, 1153-1160.

Pargament, K. (1997). *Psychology of religion and coping: Theory, research, practice.* New York: Guilford Press.

Pargament, K., Ensign, D., Falgout, K., Olsen, H., Reilly, B., Van Haitsma, K., and Warren, R. (1990). God help me (I): Religious coping efforts as predictors of the outcomes to significant negative life events. *American Journal of Community Psychology,* 18, 793-824.

Pargament, K., Kennell, J., Hathaway, W., Grevengoed, N., Newman, J., and Jones, W. (1988). Religion and the problem-solving process: Three styles of coping. *Journal for the Scientific Study of Religion,* 27(1), 90-104.

Pargament, K., Koenig, H., Tarakeshwar, N., and Hahn, J. (2001). Religious struggle as a predictor of mortality among medically ill elderly patients: A two-year longitudinal study. *Archives of Internal Medicine,* 161, 1881-1885.

Pargament, K. I. and Park, C. L. (1995). Merely a defense? The variety of religious means and ends. *Journal of Social Issues,* 51, 13-32.

Pargament, K., Smith, B., Koenig, H., and Perez, L. (1998). Patterns of positive and negative religious coping with major life stressors. *Journal for the Scientific Study of Religion,* 37(4), 710-724.

Pargament, K., Zinnbauer, B., Scott, A., Butter, E., Zerowin, J., and Stanik, P. (1998). Red flags and religious coping: Identifying some religious warning signs among people in crisis. *Journal of Clinical Psychology,* 54(1), 77-89.

Park, C. L. and Cohen, L. H. (1993). Religious and nonreligious coping with the death of a friend. *Cognitive Therapy and Research,* 17, 561-577.

Payne, E. C., Kravitz, A. R., Notman, M. T., and Anderson, J. V. (1976). Outcome following therapeutic abortion. *Archives of General Psychology,* 33, 725-733.

Propst, L. (1980). The comparative efficacy of religious and nonreligious imagery for the treatment of mild depression in religious individuals. *Cognitive Therapy and Research,* 4(2), 167-178.

Propst, L., Ostrom, P., Dean, T., and Mashburn, D. (1992). Comparative efficacy of religious and nonreligious cognitive-behavioral therapy for the treatment of clinical depression in religious individuals. *Journal of Consulting and Clinical Psychology,* 60(1), 94-103.

Rhodes, M. and Kristeller, J. (2000). The OASIS project: Oncologist-assisted spirituality intervention study. Paper presented at the annual meeting of the American Psychological Association, Washington, DC, August.

Rye, M. S. and Pargament, K. I. (2002). Forgiveness and romantic relationships in college: Can it heal the wounded heart? *Journal of Clinical Psychology,* 58(4), 419-441.

Speca, M., Carlson, L., Goodey, E., and Angen, M. (2000). A randomized, wait-listed controlled clinical trial: The effect of a mindfulnesss meditation-based stress reduction program on mood and symptoms of stress in cancer outpatients. *Psychosomatic Medicine,* 62, 613-622.

Thoresen, C. (1999). Spirituality and health: Is there a relationship? *Journal of Health Psychology,* 4(3), 291-300.

Watson, P. J., Morris, R. J., and Hood, R. W. (1988). Sin and self-functioning, part 2: Grace, guilt, and psychological adjustment. *Journal of Psychology and Theology,* 16, 270-281.

Chapter 4

Faith, Illness, and Meaning

Siroj Sorajjakool
Bryn Seyle

OBJECTIVES

1. To describe the link between existential meaning, physical illness, and spirituality. Discussion includes the human need for meaning, the search for meaning, the affect of physical illness on the personal search for meaning, and the role of spirituality and theology as they speak to the human situations of suffering and death, and also the quest for existential meaning.
2. To describe the role of faith in providing meaning to physical illness. This section discusses ways in which a person's faith in its different stages of development is related to his or her ability to find meaning in a chaotic situation, and to cope in the face of life-threatening illness and suffering.
3. To describe the role of health care professionals in providing spiritual support for patients with physical illness. This section discusses the importance of the health care professional's role in first *understanding,* and then *assisting* the patient in his or her struggle to make meaning.

INTRODUCTION

More than we may realize, illness has the potential to evoke deep theological reflection in those who are suffering. Numerous researchers have validated the relationship between religion and health, but perhaps there is more than *just* a relationship. The existential struggle with illness—especially life-threatening illness—is also a theological journey. A crisis of this kind causes us to question the previous constructs of meaning that we have given to our everyday lives. This questioning often results in a persistent search until new meaning emerges.

A couple of years ago during a group therapy session in a lockdown psychiatric unit a young woman interrupted the process with the remark, "I'm not a human being." The group counselor nodded in acknowledgment. "I really need to talk to you in private," the young woman requested.

After the session they went to a small side room. Sitting across from the counselor the young woman whispered, "I am going to tell you something really shocking."

"Tell me about it," he responded with eager anticipation.

"I plan to die on the second of June," she said. The counselor listened carefully, trying to fulfill her expectations through his expression.

"Why would you want to do that?"

"Well . . . because I'm not a human being. I'm a wolf. And I want to die so that I can become a wolf again."

The counselor pondered her statement briefly and asked how she had come to this conclusion. He wondered why she believed she was not a human being, and beyond that, why a wolf?

"I have so much pain in my life. Life is too painful. I never belong to anyone. I feel extremely sad all the time," she said.

After making another appointment to meet with her the following week the counselor still had many unanswered questions in his mind. Looking through her file he learned that she had been diagnosed with schizoaffective disorder.

During the following week's session the counselor learned about her constant feelings of sadness, her inability to get along with people, her life in a foster home, and of the aggression she was feeling. He also learned about her family's inability to take care of her. She was living by herself with her dogs—a life of sadness, loneliness, isolation, and alienation.

"What led you to think that you are a wolf and not a human being?" the counselor asked her.

"When I was little I used to have this repeating dream . . . I was howling in a cloud. I did not know why. I was rather disturbed by the dream because I did not understand its meaning. However, a couple of years later I had another dream. I dreamt that I was a little cub. I was naughty and curious. In my curiosity I left the pack and went out on my own and was killed by a wild animal. At that instant my spirit entered my dad's sperm and I became a human being."

This story may sound strange to us, but it made perfect sense to her. She needed to find an explanation for her sadness and loneliness. Having carefully thought it through, she constructed this explanation. For this young woman, having her spirit take the form of a human being was punishment for her disobedience because the human form only allowed her to feel sad and lonely. The only way she could escape this suffering was to return to her original form, the wolf. This is a very unique narration and a powerful example of the construction of meaning. Although we may find this story rather unusual, it is very common for people who face life-threatening illnesses to embark upon the process of constructing meaning to explain their situation.

MEANING AND ILLNESS

As human beings we are made for meaning, and in the presence of meaninglessness our psyches cry out, begging us to formulate an explanation that will place events in a meaningful perspective. This is especially true when individuals are confronted with a deadly illness or traumatic accident. The meaning of life seems coherent until the day when a tumor appears on the mammogram, or a car accident leads to amputation of the right leg. Then coherence turns into chaos, and one begins to question the very meaning of one's existence. Judith Herman (1992) writes, "Traumatic events overwhelm the ordinary systems of care that give people a sense of control, connection, and meaning" (p. 33). Patients often say to their counselors, "I believe God allowed this thing to happen to me," or "I believe there is a purpose for my cancer. I think God wants to use me" (or, "I think God is trying to teach me a lesson"). This need for explanation, for putting the problem into a meaningful framework, attests to the existential quest for meaning which emerges because old belief systems are no longer able to explain the present degree of suffering. Why terminal illness? Why death? What good can come out of this misery? In this experience one learns that suffering, and even the thought of death, is bearable if one is able to discover the meaning of one's existence through it. In the end it is neither death nor suffering that tortures the soul. It is the lack of meaning that becomes unbearable.

FAITH

What, then, is the place of faith when one is confronted with a life-threatening illness? The main argument of this chapter is that faith is a movement from belief in a God who intervenes by using power to heal the illness or resolve the crisis, to belief in a God who intervenes by offering comfort and courage in the time of crisis. This faith journey is comparable to the journey from childhood to adulthood. A child relies on his or her parents to take care of all of his or her needs, from breast-feeding, to bathing, to medical care, to clothing. As the child grows older the level of reliance on others to meet external needs decreases. There is movement from the parent buying the child's clothes to suggesting what the child ought to buy, from "choosing for" to teaching the child how to choose. This goes on until the individual reaches adulthood, when the child primarily depends on his or her parents for wisdom, guidance, love, and encouragement. Likewise, in the faith journey there is progression from believing in a powerful God who intervenes at every moment of our lives (stop the rain so I can go visit my girlfriend) to trust in the God who remains with us at all times as a presence of comfort and strength.

The story of the Israelites' wanderings in the wilderness for forty years offers an insight into this kind of faith transition. When the Israelites left Egypt, miracle after miracle took place for the building of their faith. The parting of the Red Sea, the pillar of fire by night and clouds by day, water coming from a rock, manna falling from heaven, and many other miraculous events were designed to teach them that God would take care of them in any situation. But before they crossed the Jordan River into Jericho an interesting event occurred.

> When the people set out from their tents to cross over the Jordan, the priests bearing the Ark of the Covenant were in front of the people. Now the Jordan overflows all its banks throughout the time of harvest. So when those who bore the ark had come to the Jordan, and the feet of the priests bearing the ark were dipped in the edge of the water, the waters flowing from above stood still, rising up in a single heap far off at Adam, the

city that is beside Zarethan, while those flowing toward the sea of the Arabah, the Dead Sea, were wholly cut off. Then the people crossed over opposite Jericho. While all Israel were crossing over on dry ground, the priests who bore the ark of the covenant of the Lord stood on dry ground in the middle of the Jordan, until the entire nation finished crossing over the Jordan. (Joshua 3:14-17, New Revised Standard Version)

Here we see how God tested the faith God had been cultivating in the Israelites. The priests did not know that the water would be parted for them. They had to step into the water and get their feet wet before they experienced the miracle. They had to make a movement from the seen into the unseen.

Perhaps the greatest example of mature faith is seen in Jesus' refusal to use external power for himself in the garden of Gethsemane or on the cross. The greatest miracle was not him "calling on ten thousand angels" for rescue, but his courage to face death at its stark worst.

The faith journey is a progressive movement to the place where one can, through God's grace, live in this sinful world of joy and misery, laughter and pain, while courageously striving to make it a better place.

FAITH AND ILLNESS

How can we relate this concept of faith to life-threatening illness? Perhaps the ideal stage for patients to be in is when they realize God's healing presence even when that which is lost may not be regained and the dying process does not cease. This concept is illustrated in the life and writings of Dietrich Bonhoeffer (1976), a German theologian who strove for justice during the Third Reich. He was hanged only a few days before the end of the war.

God is no stop-gap; he must be recognized at the centre of life, not when we are at the end of our resources; it is his will to be recognized in life, and not only when death comes; in health and vigour, and not only in suffering; in our activities, and not only in sin. The ground for this lies in the revelation of God in Jesus Christ. He is the centre of life . . . (p. 312)

As we help patients move toward the place where God becomes a source of comfort and strength to them, we must remember that it is human to struggle, and often when confronted with great distress, one will go through a stage of desperation.

Interestingly, we often shift our theological constructs in order to fit our existential struggles at the moment. We sometimes seem to regress. When faced with a crisis, there can often be a backward movement in our faith journey, but backward does not always mean negative. This is part of the rhythm of life. We grow by moving back and forth. In these crisis situations we often begin by pleading with a powerful God for a miraculous intervention. We have heard numerous stories and hope God will also intervene in our circumstances. If God does not intervene miraculously, our faith must then grow in the direction of trusting God no matter what the outcome.

An amusing and affirming incident happened to one of the church members in a local congregation. An elderly woman was admitted to the hospital. Her physician informed the church members that he did not think she had much time left. Out of concern the church elders decided to anoint her with oil, as is suggested in the Bible. The only trouble was, none of the elders had ever done this before. One Saturday afternoon six elders and the pastor walked into the patient's room with the head elder holding a bottle of olive oil in his hand. Although they had had no prior experience, most of them did not think that the entire bottle was necessary. The head elder began pouring the oil into the hands of the others. He gave each not a drop but a handful, and while praying earnestly, they all rubbed the oil onto her body. It is a bit difficult to describe her appearance after the prayer, but certainly she was one very oily patient! Amazingly, this same elderly lady is still attending church every week even though, according to her doctor's assessment, she should have passed away a year ago. Although it probably wasn't the *amount* of oil used, perhaps the volume showed how earnest those elders truly were.

Miraculous interventions are still believed to be occurring. However, it is important to have a proper perspective. There is a theological aspect to regressive behavior. According to D. W. Winnicott, regression is an indication of an inner longing for missing relational experiences (cited in Greenberg and Mitchell, 1983). Regressive behavior is an indication that we need to pay attention to our emotional reactions, in order to be able to move on to the next level of development. In a healthy relationship with God a person will go through normal developmental stages in his or her spiritual growth. In the case of faith, there seems to be a movement from belief in miraculous interventions, to acceptance of the realities of life. Regression, therefore, is a call for revision and growth in our theology, leading to a theology that imparts courage to face the raw reality of life, and to live fully every moment we have. This is where Freud went wrong. In *The Freud Reader*, Freud argued that God is a human creation, a creation that emerges out of human inability to cope with the tough reality of life. This belief may bring comfort, but to Freud, it is only an illusion.

> And thus a store of ideas is created, born from man's need to make his helplessness tolerable and built up from the material of memories of the helplessness of his own childhood and the childhood of the human race. It can clearly be seen that the possession of these ideas protects him in two directions—against the dangers of nature and Fate, and against the injuries that threaten him from human society itself. (1989, p. 695)

Perhaps in Freud's narrow interpretation of God, illusion was the only space left for God. If only he had known the God who personally suffered the appalling reality of life without interventions, the God who faced the dreadful consequences of the deliberate choice to love humankind, Freud might have come to believe that this "illusion" is indeed a reality. He might have realized that there is a God whose intervention is often one of strength and courage; a God who guides people toward maturity by offering the ability and strength to embrace life as it is. In her poem, "You Tell Me," Jewel Kilcher (1999) has painted a picture of the strong spirit of endurance that God gives to humanity.

It cannot be so
    you say
simple hands
cannot change
the fate of humanity.
        I say
Humanity is
a boundless,
absorbing heart
transcending
death and generations
and centuries
absorbing bullets
and stitches
and tear gas
enduring humiliation
and illegal abortions
and thankless jobs
        I say to you
the heart of Humanity
has not
and will not
be broken
And let us raise ourselves
like lanterns
with the millions of others—
with the mad
and the forgotten
and the strong of heart
to shine. (p. 6)

In the chaos of life when everything seems overwhelming, we may sometimes regress. Regardless, because of the human drive for existential meaning, change takes place in our interactions with God, and in our theology. There is movement toward an ever-greater understanding of God's action in our lives, and a growing faith that "accepts 'in spite of'; and out of the 'in spite of' of faith the 'in spite of' of courage is born" (Tillich, 1952, pp. 186-187). Through this development a person comes to realize that "even in the despair of having to die and the despair of self-condemnation meaning is affirmed and certitude preserved" (p. 169). This transformation often takes place in the lives of those experiencing life-threatening illnesses.

FAITH, TRANSFORMATION, AND CANCER PATIENTS

In his article, "Spirituality and the Dying Patient," Paul Rousseau (2000) states, "Every person who faces death desires that his or her life had purpose and meaning." This is because in facing death, patients are initiated into the inward journey, searching for the meaning of being, of life, and of death (Conrad, 1985).

In their qualitative research conducted at different times in two states, Patricia B. Fryback and Bonita Reinert (1999) interviewed fifteen individuals. Ten were women with cancer and the rest were men with HIV/AIDS. The primary purpose was to find out how these individuals with terminal diagnoses viewed and experienced the concept of health. Results showed that all fifteen participants identified spirituality as the primary component of health. Three concepts identified were: belief in a higher power, recognition of mortality, and self-actualization. Of interest is the relationship between meaning and spirituality. "Finding meaning is particularly important when a person is facing a serious illness, because the illness itself causes permanent changes in life that force a reevaluation of any previously assumed meaning" (p. 20). Or as one of the participants said, "health has more to do with some sort of spiritual foundation" than with physical issues (p. 20). People who found meaning through their illnesses believed that there was more quality in their lives than prior to their diagnosis (Fryback and Reinhart, 1999).

A qualitative study by Joan Thomas and Andrew Retsas (1999) showed similar results. They interviewed nineteen patients with terminal cancer who were living in Queensland and New South Wales, Australia. The aim of this study was to explain how the spirituality of terminal cancer patients played a role in making sense of, and coming to terms with their diagnosis. They found that people with terminal cancer developed spiritual perspectives that strengthened their approaches to life and death. This was accomplished through the process of transacting self-preservation, which incorporates three phases: taking it all in, getting on with things, and putting it all together. This process dramatically aids the understanding of self. It also enhances spiritual growth, spiritual perspective, spiritual awareness, and spiritual experience.

A study by Siroj Sorajjakool and Bryn Seyle (2003) on the relationship between illness and meaning among cancer patients offered interesting insights regarding changes in theological perspective that enabled these patients to cope better with their life-threatening illnesses. Some of these insights are summarized as follows:

1. Cancer is a catalyst for change in a person's theology. How an individual perceives God and God's involvement in his or her life is strongly affected by illness.

   I think visually I had thought of God as being up there and perhaps . . . distant but not real distant, and providing support, kind of, from up there. . . . I have much more of a sense of God now being beneath me, holding me up, supporting me in a much more direct fashion than I had had before. . . . It's a different perspective for me.

An Asian economic journalist expressed how cancer had transformed her theology:

   Every time you go through that experience [cancer] your values change, and your perspective on life changes so the worldview is different.

2. Those who accept cancer as a part of their reality (their worldview) have less difficulty dealing with the disease. This became apparent in talking with the interviewees. One woman said that her friends spent more time trying to figure out why this was happening to her than she did.

   I don't think it was an act of God . . . nor was it anything personal. And when I look back I don't think there was anything I could have done otherwise to have prevented it. . . .What else I could have done differently, I don't know. It could have been genetic . . . it was just one of those things. . . . To me cancer doesn't discriminate between race, sex, religion . . . the young, the poor. . . . It happened and I accepted it, and I guess I just want to move on more than anything else. I just don't want to waste too much time and energy trying to figure it out. . . . It's like one of those profound things in life like "why am I here, what is the purpose of my life."

It seems that those individuals who had previously experienced a major loss or illness, and thus viewed cancer as something that could happen to anyone, were more likely to accept their illness as a part of reality.

I think prior to my diagnosis of cancer I knew that bad things happen to good people, and I had experiences in my childhood with losing my father, losing my brother at a young age and seeing other family members go through very difficult things. . . . Prior to my diagnosis of cancer I watched my mother-in-law who I think is just one of the most wonderful saintly Christian women in the world, go through a horrible experience with cancer, and I guess I had to reconcile some of those issues of why bad things happened at that point . . . and again I came to the point of feeling that this was not something that God wanted, this was not something that God caused but there is evil in the world, and that this is a consequence of evil in the world.

3. Individuals who believe that everything happens for a reason, and that God is in charge of every occurrence in life have a more difficult time accepting their illness.

A female health care worker with breast cancer who had struggled harder than some of the other patients in coming to terms with her diagnosis explained why she thought this was happening to her:

A wake-up call, you know . . . to appreciate life more, to have a stronger relationship with God, to have the experience behind me to help other people, to somehow touch somebody's life in my future and help them with what I've learned. Who knows, maybe I'll be able to contribute somehow to decreasing breast cancer in the future . . . somehow there is a reason why I've gone through this. . . . I really did not expect to have cancer, I always thought that it was . . . somebody else. I would never get cancer.

Another breast cancer patient who experienced recurring depression annually at the time of her diagnosis stated:

When the word cancer hits you, when they pronounce cancer . . . that word had a big impact. First when I heard that I just denied. More than 100 percent . . . one thing that I realized—I never questioned God, why me? That's the thing . . . I count my blessings, I never questioned God. But just denied it, it cannot be me. But when you hear that, how can you cope with it? . . . All you do is just deny and be angry.

After recovering from breast cancer one client says that her God no longer remains in the box she had constructed for him; he works in mysterious ways, and she no longer tells him what to do or what she thinks he ought to do. She now lets God be God.

SPIRITUAL CARE

How then, can we as caregivers provide spiritual care for individuals in their times of crisis? We need to pay attention to the soul. Regarding the care of the soul Thomas Moore (1992) states:

Care of the soul speaks to the longings we feel and to the symptoms that drive us crazy, but it is not a path away from shadow or death. A soulful personality is complicated, multifaceted, and shaped by both pain and pleasure, success and failure. Life lived soulfully is not without its moments of darkness and periods of foolishness. Dropping the salvation fantasy frees us up to the possibility of self-knowledge and self-acceptance, which are the very foundation of soul. (pp. xvi-xvii)

Often there are inexplicable mysteries in life, times when there seems to be no logic or rationality in events. How do we bring grace to individuals who are faced with the disruption of their lives through the experience of cancer or other debilitating illnesses? How do we help them construct meaning in the face of death? The answer is love. The apostle Paul wrote, "And now faith, hope, and love abide. But the greatest of these is love" (1 Corinthians 13:13).

Unconditional love is the power that enables a person to tolerate the chaos when things do not seem to make sense. Love adds meaning to the irrational, creates sense for the nonsensical. It defies logic by making pain endurable. It is the only source of meaning in the face of meaninglessness. It explains when nothing else makes sense. Meaning is not derived primarily by the rational mind putting all the pieces of the puzzle of life together. Meaning is an existential journey of the heart. Meaning comes about when one is able to tolerate the irrational turmoil of pain while resting in the embrace of love.

Perhaps this is why sick people come to the hospital. It is a place of hospitality, a place that offers the embrace of illness in the presence of care. "The word *hospital,*" writes Moore (1992), "comes from *hospis,* which means both 'stranger' and 'host,' plus *pito,* meaning 'lord' or 'powerful one.' The hospital is a place where the stranger can find rest, protection, and care" (p. 175). If patients are given only cold uncaring treatment, even though the latest equipment and therapies are used, and experience no love or compassionate concern from medical caregivers during their hospital stay, they will not really have gotten the rest, protection, and care a hospital should provide for them.

The experience of meaning may not mean making rational sense of illness or finding an explanation for the problem of suffering. Meaning can take place at the existential level, which can perhaps transcend the rational. This offering of meaning in a concrete way is not achieved through the process of interpretation, theological explanation, or philosophical reflection. Love is experienced at the existential level, when one's story, one's struggle, is being heard in a real way. This is the offering of love that creates meaning in the midst of chaos, clearing a space and allowing internal thoughts, feelings, struggles, hurt, and confusion to emerge and to be recognized. This act of love calls only for space, time, and the willingness to listen attentively. Through the experience of love, a hurting patient knows that although the pain and chaos may remain, his or her life takes on a new meaning.

CONCLUSION

When faced with a major crisis, individuals question who they are. The instinctive response is an engagement in the quest that leads ultimately to the incorporation of this new experience into a belief system that makes sense. Often the primary response is to remain within the previously held belief system. However, it is important to recognize that life crisis, in some ways, is an invitation to another level in faith development. This is the movement from the belief in a miraculous intervention to the place where we come to see God as a God whose presence remains with us throughout our pain, our journey. As caregivers, it is critical to create a safe space in which the transition from one stage of faith to the next can take place. The caring and listening presence of caregivers can offer help in finding that new meaning; the existential understanding that it is all right to feel the anger, chaos, frustration, and pain. This new meaning through the listening presence helps people realize that while things may not make sense, God remains. The touch of love offers meaning that transcends understanding and explanation.

John Schumacher (1998) wrote a short story that illustrates the place and the power of love in the ministry of healing: There was a little girl who watched her grandmother dying. The experience raised many questions about death, loss, and God in her mind. Her mother told her that the chaplain would come and answer all her questions. In her excitement she wrote them all down. When the chaplain came he noticed the little girl sitting across from him, surrounded by her family. Slowly she began to read her questions to him. She sat quietly listening to each answer, and then read her next question. The chaplain knew that his answers were not sufficient, that no one could definitively answer her questions. So he affirmed her questions, let her know that her feelings were important, and offered her the assurance that her family loved her so much that they wanted to hear all her questions, even though they were hard to answer.

> Finally, the child stopped questioning and began to cry. Perhaps she cried in frustration because the adults had no answers, or in fear from an experience she could not understand, or in sadness at her grandmother's dying. Most certainly she cried because she knew she was surrounded by people who loved her, and it was safe to cry.
>
> And many other people in that kitchen felt free to cry with her, some for the first time since they were told that grandmother would die. (p. 191)

GUIDED QUESTIONS

1. How does illness affect a sense of meaning among patients who have been diagnosed with serious illness?
2. What changes usually occur in the journey of faith?
3. What role does regression play in one's theological construction?
4. Discuss findings of Patricia B. Fryback and Bonita Reinert in relation to breast cancer patients.
5. What role does love play in the process of meaning making?

REFERENCES

Bonhoeffer, Dietrich (1976). *Letters and papers from prison.* New York: Macmillan.

Conrad, N. L. (1985). Spiritual support for the dying. *Nurses Clinic in North America,* 20, 415-426.

Freud, Sigmund (1989). *The Freud reader,* Peter Gay, ed. New York: W. W. Norton and Company.

Fryback, Patricia and Reinert, Bonita (1999). Spirituality and people with potentially fatal diagnoses. *Nursing Forum,* 34(1), 13-22.

Greenberg, Jay R. and Mitchell, Stephen A. (1983). *Object relations in psychoanalytic theory.* Cambridge, MA: Harvard University Press.

Herman, Judith (1992). *Trauma and recovery: The aftermath of violence from domestic abuse to political terrors.* New York: BasicBooks.

Kilcher, Jewel (1999). *A night without armor.* New York: HarperEntertainment.

Moore, Thomas (1992). *Care of the soul: A guide for cultivating depth and sacredness in everday life.* New York: HarperPerennial.

Rousseau, Paul (2000). Spirituality and the dying patient: The art of oncology: When the tumor is not the target. *Journal of Clinical Oncology,* 18(9), 2000-2002.

Schumacher, John E. (1998). Unless you become as little children . . . *Journal of Pastoral Care,* 52(2), 191.

Sorajjakool, Siroj and Seyle, Bryn (2003). Impact of illness on theological constructs among cancer patients. Unpublished paper.

Thomas, Joan and Retsas, Andrew (1999). Transacting self-preservation: A grounded theory of the spiritual dimensions of people with terminal cancer. *International Journal of Nursing Studies,* 36, 191-201.

Tillich, Paul (1952). *Courage to be.* Glasgow: Collins.

PART II:
PRAXIS

Chapter 5

Spiritual Care: Basic Principles

James Greek

OBJECTIVES

1. To define spiritual care from an integrated perspective and increase the understanding of health care professionals on how to make meaningful emotional, spiritual, and physical connections with patients.
2. To describe the basic premise, purpose, and process of spiritual care.
3. To outline key components to increase the efficacy of spiritual caregiving.
4. To provide a learning tool, specific to health care providers, for addressing the importance of spiritual contributions to overall health care.

INTRODUCTION

The maiden voyage of the *Titanic* left promptly at noon on April 10, 1912. There were 2,228 passengers and crew. The ship was approximately three football fields in length and more like a floating palace than a boat. The first-class smoking section had carved mahogany woodwork inlaid with mother-of-pearl, and the furniture had dark green leather upholstery. At that time it was the largest moving object ever made by man.

The passengers represented a cross section of humanity determined to enjoy this historic trip to the fullest. There were common citizens, the wealthy, the famous, and the media. It was a festive occasion with the band playing favorite contemporary musical numbers. All was safe and predictable until the iceberg made contact.

In the midst of the ensuing chaos in which only 705 souls were saved, witnesses tell that the band kept playing but changed from popular music to "Nearer My God to Thee." How true it is that often in life, crises bring us back to the spiritual.

As a method of dealing with life, individuals often wrap their identities around their success, wealth, prestige, family, or accomplishments. Then a crisis hits and they find themselves in the hospital waiting for the results of medical tests. In these vulnerable moments the things that once brought comfort lose their power. Many feel a need for greater help—help from outside themselves. Here we enter the world of "spiritual care."

Within the concept of "wholeness," the "spiritual" is a foundational component. Current research demonstrates that spiritual support definitely affects both emotional and physical healing.

Spiritual care is not a nebulous, touchy-feely concept in which we psyche ourselves up to live another day. It represents the stirring truth that we are not alone as individuals or humankind. The record of God's creation of humans reads, "Let us make man in our own image, after our likeness" (Genesis 1:26). There is a link between the human and the spiritual. The spiritual is a part of who we are, integral to our wholeness and healing. Without this dimension we experience brokenness.

When the Israelites were in the wilderness God gave Moses instructions to "make me a sanctuary; that I may dwell among them" (Exodus 25:8). This tent was located in the middle of their encampment, signifying God's place in their affairs. It was God's desire to be with the people as they journeyed through the desert. It was God's plan to be a source of strength and encouragement as they faced the challenges along the way. The underlying premise of spiritual care is that God still takes an interest in the plight of people. Although miraculous intervention may not take place, there is always the promise of presence, encouragement, and strength to face the future.

Several years ago my wife and I traveled across the beautiful state of New Mexico. As we came over a small hill we were astonished to see giant antenna dishes spread out over miles of desert. They seemed to cover the entire desert floor. Our curiosity was piqued, so we stopped to ask the purpose of this array of technology. We found we had stumbled upon a group belonging to an organization called SETI—people who search for extraterrestrial life. They were listening for a phone call from space.

In providing spiritual care it is our privilege to strengthen the link between the patient and his or her spiritual resources. This is not a phone call from outer space, but a connection that brings comfort and strength from a real God to a real person in need.

Several years ago a patient came into my life that forever instilled in me the power and significance of the spiritual in facing crisis. I'll call him Steve. It was approximately 2:00 p.m. when I received a page to the trauma unit. A patient had recently been flown in by helicopter and was in serious condition. However, this was only the tip of the iceberg.

Before entering the room I was briefed by the medical staff. There had been an automobile accident involving not only the patient but also his wife and twin girls. Sadly, his wife and one of the twins had died. The second little girl was in serious condition. Steve had sustained a broken neck and would probably be quadriplegic the rest of his life.

With this background I was asked to speak with Steve. Though I had visited thousands of patients in the past, no experience could compare with this man's loss. As I entered the room I noticed the metal halo covering his head. Though awake he seemed to be staring off into space. I could only imagine the intensity of his emotions and did not know what to expect from him.

Because he could not move his head I positioned myself looking down into his halo and face. I told him softly that I was the chaplain and was profoundly sorry for his loss. His eyes looked deeply into mine, and after a moment of silence he spoke in a whisper, "Chaplain, I just lost my soul mate. She was the love of my life. My little girl is dead. My other daughter is alive but will probably be handicapped the rest of her life. I will never hold them again in this life. I recently completed four years of computer training but will never touch a computer again. God . . . God did not do this. But because of God I believe I will see my family again one day. I know he [God] will help me go on with life, as painful as it is." He then turned his face from me and looked up at the ceiling. I knew he wasn't speaking to me any longer when he said, "Naked came I into this world and naked I will leave. Blessed be the name of the Lord" (Job 1:21).

I visited Steve many times after this first visit. There were sessions with tears and at times great anguish. However, his faith in God remained and was a source of strength far beyond what I had ever witnessed before.

Steve had a strong personal faith before this tragedy. His spiritual resources had been clearly defined in his own mind. Unfortunately this is not so in every case. In delivering spiritual care it is important to recognize that people are at different stages of spiritual growth though they may have similar spiritual needs.

Spiritual care is not reserved for certain individuals, belief systems, churches, or denominations. It does not matter if a person is a Protestant, Catholic, Muslim, Hindu, or any other religion we might name, or no religion, even agnostic or atheist. Because we are all part of humanity we experience the same needs. Therefore it is important to respect each person's faith position while attempting to meet their needs. *Spiritual care occurs when the caregiver takes the initiative to enter another's world for the purpose of discerning current needs. These needs may include the physical, emotional, and/or spiritual areas of life. Spiritual resources to address those needs are then explored with the patient.*

Though a "patient visit" is not a hard science, there are dynamics involved that give direction to the caregiver. Creation of a trusting atmosphere, evaluation of the patient, listening skills, identifying with humanness, prayer, the caregiver's own heart preparation, etc., are all components affecting the spiritual care process. The remainder of this chapter discusses twelve suggestions for helping caregivers accomplish their important goals in their patient visits.

TWELVE SUGGESTIONS FOR A SPIRITUAL VISIT

Know Thyself

Spiritual care does not happen in a vacuum. It takes a real warm-blooded person to touch another warm-blooded person who happens to be in need. In this contact spiritual care is either communicated or not.

Much of what we bring to the patient's bedside begins in the heart of the one bringing the care. As we ponder the task and opportunity of providing help on a spiritual level, we may hear a call beckoning us to seek solitude for the work of our own personal preparation. The caregiver's words and influence will exude sincerity that will be perceived by the patient when that caregiver has, through personal experience, reached the awareness and conviction that spiritual care does in fact make a difference in patients' lives.

One morning I accompanied the plastic surgery team on their patient rounds. The team leader asked a patient where she received strength to face her medical problem. The response surprised some of us. She said, "I get my strength from the eyes of the physician." In the eyes of the physician she perceived that she was more than "just another patient." She felt she was viewed as a human being deserving respect and genuine care. This level of caring requires frequent solitude to reflect, maintain, and deepen our concern and love for those in our care. Without charging our own spiritual batteries regularly we may be in danger of losing compassion—the very heart of spiritual care.

Balance is also important for caregivers. We can offer spiritual and emotional support and encourage patients in their struggle. But ultimately how the patient decides to cope depends on him or her alone. In his book *Good Intentions,* Duke Robinson states:

> The key to serving others will be your willingness and ability to back off from trying to resolve what besets them. This is not a matter of turning your back on your friends or refusing to listen to them. It is not asking you to create emotional distance from them as persons, to be partially present to them or not present at all when they need you the most. It simply asks you not to assume responsibility for their lives. (1997, pp. 183-184)

Create a Safe Atmosphere

In providing spiritual care it is extremely important to recognize the dynamics of the patient/caregiver relationship. For many patients the beeps, buzzes, smells, tubes, flashing lights, codes, and so on, create an atmosphere of vulnerability or downright fear. It is a world many cannot interpret, where imagination may be the worst enemy. A young military man and I were conversing about his future when one of the machines next to his bed began to beep and flash red. He told me that when this happens he feels like diving into a foxhole. With his anxiety level already high, he interpreted every unusual sound as "something must be going wrong with me." Hospital stays are fraught with feelings of loss of control. This is the setting, however, that the caregiver needs to be aware of in attempting to create a safe environment for patients.

From the moment we enter the room the patient begins an evaluation of us. Can there be sufficient trust for weary souls to unfold the deep underlying issues? Dan Allender states that "it is God's passionate business to send us into the stories of others" (1999, p. 222). We are entering onto the holy ground of others' lives.

Through experience and observation of mentors I have found some simple but important tips for creating a "safe environment" to enhance the effectiveness of a spiritual visit.

Personal demeanor sets the stage for communication. If I appear rushed or look like I am attempting to cover my "twenty questions" as quickly as possible in order to move on to the next patient, I will send the message that the information I seek is more important than the person I am standing before. A telephone company once conducted a survey to stay competitive. It found that when its operators spoke calmly and slowly, credibility went up in customers' minds. Likewise, though our visit may be short, our calmness of speech and caring tones will build trust and open doors to deeper issues.

Focus is another important consideration. Several years ago I attended a conference for approximately 15,000 professionals. Greeters were out in force to welcome the invitees. As I entered the main auditorium a greeter took my hand and uttered the words, "It's so wonderful to have you here for this great occasion. I know you will enjoy your stay and gather a wealth of information." Her words were very appropriate and should have made me feel welcome. However, this was not the case. While she was welcoming me, her face was turned to my right and she was waving at her friends as they walked by. It appeared that she was simply going through the routine of greeting without real sincerity. In the midst of her waving I asked where the men's room was located and she said "yes."

Focusing on the patient simply means he or she experiences your availability both verbally and nonverbally. This can be conveyed through eye contact, touching, sitting down in a chair so your eyes are on the same level, the direction of your body, tones of voice, etc.

Some people may be concerned about touching and the issue of sexual harassment. However, simply placing one's hand on the patient's forearm conveys the message of unhurried care. In Mark 5:25-31 Jesus walks down the road with a crowd of people. Jesus asks, "Who touched me?" A disciple implies that many people are touching him. However, Jesus makes the point that there is a difference between the common touch and the touch of caring. As health care givers much of our work involves touching people. The patients know the difference between us doing our job and the special touch given for emotional/spiritual support. Establishing a safe atmosphere creates a setting where this goal becomes a possibility.

Be Aware of Your Surroundings

What is meant by being aware of your surroundings in the context of spiritual care? At times it may seem challenging to enter the room of a stranger and later walk away with intimate information regarding his or her faith and religious resources. However, there are points of contact you can look for that will aid you in entering into patients' lives. When visiting patients with fourth-year medical students I share the importance of scanning the room with "spiritual care eyes" as they enter the door. What are we looking for? Avenues to the soul. One will often find simple objects like flowers, pictures, books, trinkets, etc., that can be used by the caregiver to enter the life of the patient. When we see flowers on the stand and take time to find out who sent them, a wealth of personal information often flows. Taking an interest in family pictures identifies the support the patient is receiving and often ties you closer to the patient in preparation for discussion of deeper spiritual issues. A Bible, cross, or other religious material belonging to the patient can springboard you into questions of his or her spiritual resources.

Being aware of your surroundings can give you instant direction before the first word is even spoken.

Identify with the Patient's Humanness

George was a thirty-five-year-old construction worker who was hurt while digging a trench. His spiritual background was very limited, and he appeared uncomfortable when he realized I was a chaplain. The first visit was short and the second visit appeared to be headed for a quick end as well. He did not want to talk. As the conversation began to close I noticed a picture of George holding up a rainbow trout. I paused a moment and said, "You know, George, I grew up in Florida and we caught big mouth bass but I've always wondered what it would be like to catch trout." In the next five minutes I received an interesting talk on what it was like to catch trout. After he finished he said, "You know, chaplain . . . I'm scared. But I'm not sure how to talk to God." We had a meaningful and helpful time of sharing. He later told me, "I'm nervous around preachers or those who might try to convert me. But when you showed an interest in the things I am interested in I felt myself open up. It made me," he continued, "feel like I wasn't talking to someone who feels superior to me or even judgmental. I was talking to another human being who has similar interests."

Since that visit years ago I have found myself speaking with patients about their dogs, skiing, camping, cooking, cars, etc., as I make the journey to their hearts. It is okay to be human with people.

Let the Patient Be Your Teacher

After a safe environment is created the caregiver will often find that conversation and information about the patient's life will flow freely. As trained professionals with years of experience and skill in verbalizing our thoughts, we may be tempted to dominate the conversation. Some people are so apt in their communication abilities that they have learned to manipulate feelings by saying the right things in the right way at the right time! An individual from another medical institution told me that he felt so confident in his "people skills" that he could go into anyone's hospital room and make them feel better. The patient's issues may not have been dealt with but he or she would "feel better," at least for a little while.

True spiritual care involves much more than superficially making people feel better. True spiritual care—helping people get in touch with and utilize to the fullest their own spiritual resources—comes from identifying the issues causing their pain, whether emotional or physical, and then bathing them in the patient's faith and the caregiver's spiritual support. In order for this to happen we must let patients teach us about themselves.

During the conversation the caregiver should be attentive to information that surfaces which may be considered a "red flag." In other words, specific issues may come up that constitute sources of pain, anxiety, and concern. These issues may greatly affect the patient's ability to cope with his or her medical challenges. Here are some examples of "red flag" situations.

Susan was in the ICU after a serious automobile accident. Fortunately, after the tests were completed it was determined that she had only suffered a broken leg and a mild concussion. Though uncomfortable, she would be back to normal soon. This should have been good news, but Susan remained in a depressed state for days. Though compliant with the physician's instructions, she reflected a deep sense of hopelessness. During the first two visits she gave short answers that revealed little. On the third visit she stated in almost a whisper, "I miss John." Immediately she caught herself and tried to change the subject. Here was a "red flag." I asked softly, "Who is John?" She looked up as the tears began to flow and said, "John was my brand-new husband. He was killed one month ago in a job-related accident. He was all I had and I loved him deeply." The broken leg and mild concussion were of little consequence compared to the grief she was experiencing beneath the surface.

Elizabeth's surgery appeared to be a success. The mastectomy had been completed and the cancer was removed. To all outward appearances she was coping well. Though she asked all the right questions, the physician sensed concern in her eyes. Because the physician believed in healing the whole person he took their conversations seriously. Thinking back, he realized she had never brought up the subject of her husband. One day he asked the question, "How is Jim handling your surgery?" She flinched, looked down, and after an eternity of silence said, "Doctor, I think Jim is having trouble accepting me as a whole woman now that I have had this surgery. I am more afraid of the loss of his love than the cancer."

Tony lay in a hospital bed with a bullet hole in his shoulder—the result of gang activity in the area. Though young in age, his face revealed the stresses of survival on the street. After a number of visits Tony felt safe in saying that he wanted out of gang life. We began thinking of ways to enroll him in a vocational program. At times he was positive, but then for no apparent reason he would swing into a state of deep guilt. After approximately four more visits I asked him to speak of his past. He stated, "I think I stabbed another gang member with my knife years ago. I think it was serious but I never read about it in the newspaper. Because of this I have no right to enjoy life myself."

What do all these stories have in common? Each patient eventually taught us where their deepest issues were. This awareness directed our ministry to them, and helped us "hit the target" where the real issues were. To have a focused spiritual ministry we must listen and let the patient be our teacher.

Ask Well-Chosen Questions

During visits some patients feel free to volunteer important information that will guide the caregiver. However, others may feel awkward in conversation, thus presenting a challenge to the one conducting the visit. It is important to determine as accurately as possible where the patient is emotionally and spiritually in life in general and in his or her current medical situation. With this information one can tailor questions to the patient's needs rather than simply entering into a generic conversation hoping that something will "turn up."

Years ago I played on a college tennis team in Florida. We had a great coach who wore us out in our afternoon practice sessions. One day before an important match with a top-notch team he gathered our team together and said, "I have one bit of counsel to give you that will make you victors." We were all ears as he made his big pronouncement: "If you want to win, hit the ball where your opponent is not." It wasn't the most profound statement our coach had ever made, but it was true!

The same truth applies in reverse for facilitating a conversation with a patient. To reach the heart of the patient direct your questions to where the patient *is*.

For example, if working with an individual who was recently told he has six months to live it would seem appropriate to focus questions on end-of-life issues. For example, how does he plan on spending the remainder of his life? Does he want to focus on the disease or spend remaining moments in quality time with loved ones? If the patient is open to spiritual things, focused questions could direct him toward spiritual preparation for death.

John was in the ICU as the result of an automobile accident in which he lost his leg. On the table was a picture of his wife and three little girls. He was in his mid-thirties and did physical labor for his life's work. During the visit John was cordial but quiet. After evaluating his situation I asked him, "Are you worried about how you will support your wife and little girls now?" The medical staff watched as a tear trickled down his cheek. He said, "I have always cared for and protected my family, but how can I do it now?"

It was more than a leg; it was John's identity that was "lost," at least in his mind. His ability to care for those he loved most was threatened and he was experiencing fear. In future visits he confided that he also wondered if his wife could love "half a man."

As is the case with many patients, John could not see beyond the box he was in. All he could think of was the crisis of his present experience. During initial visits he even expressed anger toward God for "letting this happen."

How does one deliver spiritual care in a setting such as this? First, spiritual care is not a "magic bullet" or a quick fix. Receptivity to spiritual care is often determined by the readiness of the patient to accept spiritual overtures offered by the caregiver.

John's fears, anger, and questionings represent the experience of many others impacted by trauma. It can be an intense time of self-expression. What John needed was someone to listen even for a few moments. Someone to acknowledge his fears and his loss . . . someone to say it is okay to be afraid . . . it is okay to be angry and to even question God.

Through dialogue with the caregiver, John became less reactive and more rational. Was he still under stress? Yes. But the emotional paralysis resulting from the trauma slowly subsided and he began to see life a little clearer.

As the days progressed he was open to discuss his views on God's role in the accident. The caregiver asked "John, after having a few days to think about it, how does God fit into your life right now?" He stated, "My knee-jerk reaction was that God did this to me. However, after thinking more I realize that God was not driving the car . . . a drunk was. God is not in the business of hurting people." Slowly his faith once again became a positive resource for his present dilemma.

Had the caregiver attempted to defend God or correct the patient's views on the initial visit future dialogue on spiritual issues could have been hampered.

Drawing on the spiritual commitment from his wife and church the patient became convinced that he would not face the future alone. Though there would be lifestyle changes he was at peace that his family was committed to reinventing the future together.

Though other stories may not always turn out as positive, asking appropriate questions helps patients not only to feel understood but also brings them into contact with their real needs. This gives direction to and opportunity for spiritual care.

What does all this have to do with spiritual care? Spiritual care is not standing at the end of a bed with a Bible like a televangelist, attempting to influence the patient into making a decision. Spiritual care is coming close to the heart of patients so we become aware of their burdens, both above and below the surface.

When this happens, and trust develops between the patient and caregiver, it becomes natural to discuss the patient's spiritual resources. If the patient believes you really care for his or her plight you will often find the "door open."

How do you broach the topic of spirituality with a patient? Many are hesitant to enter this dialogue for fear of offending the patient. I have found that a more casual approach is less offensive and easier for the one asking the question. Instead of asking, "Do you go to church?" or "Do you believe in God?" I have asked, "In light of all you are going through, where do you get your strength to cope? What do you depend on?" Sometimes they will say "family," but more often they will say "prayer," "God," or even point up to heaven. When patients respond in this manner it gives you permission to ask questions about spiritual resources because they have volunteered the fact that they believe in God. This approach gives patients the choice to allow you into this part of their private life. It respects the patient.

Mirror What You Hear

Being understood is power in a conversation. In our fast-paced society the temptation is to gather the information and depart. Whole-person care, particularly the spiritual aspects, requires the touching of life with life, soul with soul. For that to occur the patient needs to feel understood. Being understood in the common areas of life allows us to delve into the more private spiritual areas.

While participating on rounds with the plastic surgery team I witnessed a patient being understood. The physician conducting the rounds was surrounded with approximately six students and the chaplain. As we entered the room I noticed the patient had tubes in his mouth. Though fully alert he could not communicate verbally. The physician wanted the students to understand the history and concerns of the patient. Without notes or a chart the physician walked us through the man's family and medical history. He spoke of the patient's little son and daughter and how he longed to go home. He then reflected on the patient's spiritual resources with the Catholic church and the good support he was receiving from his family. The doctor also expressed the patient's fears accurately. The patient's eyes were locked on the physician as he spoke. Unsolicited, he reached out and squeezed the doctor's hand. Later, the family said their loved one felt like we really understood his plight because of the way the physician summarized his situation for the students.

Many people are not used to facing how they feel, so they mask their feelings or portray a strong front. When someone can verbalize their true feelings or fears for them, it helps them more readily accept what they are experiencing, and ushers them along the path toward emotional and spiritual healing.

Being understood sends a message that we are not alone. Someone else knows what we are going through. As whole-person care representatives it is our privilege to enter other people's lives. By mirroring their journey during the conversation, doors will open to address spiritual issues, and as the bond grows between the patient and caregiver opportunities may arise to share our own spiritual resources with the patient. This reminds me of a story about the apostle Peter. Peter said to a man who had been crippled from birth, "Silver or gold I do not have, but what I have I give you" (Acts 3:6). We may not be able to cure the sickness of patients, but we may find an opportunity to connect them to spiritual resources that will help to heal their outlook on life in spite of their illness.

Reevaluate a Patient's Spiritual Status

Many of us are well-informed regarding the ongoing debates centering on evolution and Darwinism. Lines have been drawn for years around the micro and macro aspects of change within species and between species. No matter what one feels about this topic, the truth is that evolution of a spiritual nature often occurs in hospital beds throughout the world.

Elizabeth entered the hospital with necrotizing fasciitis disease (a type of flesh-eating disease). She was a strong Christian who regularly attended a Protestant church in the Los Angeles area. During our first visit she conveyed that her faith would "see me through."

Her husband was present for family and spiritual support. As far as we could ascertain, her support systems were firmly in place. During future visits we were confident she was handling her challenges well.

However, as her stay lengthened and her physical condition showed little sign of improvement, her efforts to "hold on to her faith" intensified. There was now an air of desperation in her voice, though this would be natural for anyone in her situation. Her faith was being shaken. After two weeks her questions began: "Is God testing me?" "Did I do something to displease him?" Finally, she reached the conclusion that God did not care for her and had in fact abandoned her. She even began entertaining the possibility that God did not exist.

These questions often arise when people struggle with trauma regardless of their religious beliefs. Some people's faith grows stronger under trial but others struggle. Caregivers should not rely only on the first spiritual evaluation, especially if the patient's stay is prolonged or his or her condition deteriorates.

In his book, *When Bad Things Happen to Good People,* Harold Kushner addresses the haunting question that caregivers and patients often contemplate.

> There is only one question which really matters: why do bad things happen to good people? All other theological conversation is intellectually diverting; somewhat like doing the cross-

word puzzle in the Sunday paper and feeling very satisfied when
you have made the words fit; but ultimately without the capacity
to reach people where they really care. (1981, p. 6)

People tend to reevaluate the reality of their faith in the midst of
trial. This phenomenon needs to be understood by caregivers if we
are to bring real spiritual support to them on their journey. Therefore,
it is important to take a "reading" of their status periodically. Questions such as, "Are you able to maintain your hold on God when
things don't make sense?" may be asked. Another question could be,
"It is obvious you have been going through a great deal these past
weeks. How is your faith holding up?"

Only the patient can wrestle with his or her own faith, but having
an interested party to discuss it with is helpful. Though the dynamics
of this are not fully understood, emotional and spiritual healing often
follows telling our stories.

False ideas and misconceptions often exacerbate this shaking of
the patient's faith. Patients may believe that bad things occur as a consequence of their misdeeds. Or, they may feel that God will always
heal us if our faith is strong enough. They conclude when they are not
healed, that their faith must be inadequate. Misconceptions such as
these can cause a great deal of distress.

Also complicating the process may be the patient's grief over losing his or her independence, function, or even limbs. Friends who
gave initial support may begin to drift away because they have run out
of things to say and feel ineffective. All these issues affect spiritual
endurance. Caregivers should take "spiritual checks" along the way
to evaluate patients' levels of spirituality.

Anyone Can Pray

Prayer is the universal language experienced in common between
systems of beliefs. In other words, no matter what belief one holds,
prayer is at the heart of it. This means prayer can be an effective
means to spiritually strengthen patients.

People in hospitals tend to be more open to spiritual care. Though
they may not regularly pray in their private lives, many have learned
about prayer at their mother's knee, or from a spiritual relative or ac-
quaintance. Rarely have I had patients refuse to be prayed for. The
real question is when and how to pray.

The timing of prayer is very important. If one follows the earlier steps of creating a safe environment, taking an interest in the patient as a person, etc., prayer becomes a natural follow-through. Prayer is most effective when we know the person. Trust is built and doors are opened to enter into the deeper recesses of the patient's life.

However, it is amazing how quickly a caring relationship can develop on the first visit. Taking an interest in an individual has more to do with quality of interaction than the amount of time spent or number of visits. I have observed physicians enter a patient's life and participate in prayer on the very first visit. This is important for the doctor who sees the patient for only one time.

The second consideration regarding prayer is how to pray. When I go with medical students on rounds I will sometimes ask them to pray. The natural question arises, "What do I pray for?" Many of us have learned rote prayers passed down from generation to generation. However, what patients most need through the medium of prayer is communication with God about their current intense needs. I share with students that during the conversation I make a mental note of areas of concern the patient reveals and pray for these needs.

Though God knows every person's plight, there is healing in hearing those needs expressed audibly to God in the presence of the patient, even if by a stranger.

Sometimes, patients appear emotionally detached until prayer is offered—then the walls come down. Prayer interfaces us with our inner selves. Praying specifically for the patient's needs is something anyone can do and the results can be powerful. Do not be deceived by a patient's appearance or attitude. Most patients feel the need for sincere prayer and need someone bold enough to ask, "May I pray for you?"

Be a Person of Hope

As mentioned earlier, a patient was asked, "Where do you get your hope?" The patient immediately responded, "In the eyes of my doctor." In a recent lecture the speaker stated that when laughter is present endorphins increase, thus strengthening the immune system. The implication was that external stimuli could affect healing. The lecturer then posed for consideration the idea that how we as medical staff approach and interact with patients may one day be proven to impact healing and health. Do we approach patients with hope or emotional neutrality that can be interpreted as hopelessness?

Does this mean we should be in the business of giving hope when there is no reason to hope? Should we peddle a false type of security? The answer is a resounding no. But there is a hope that transcends being cured. It is the hope that remains in the presence of adversity.

It is possible to be healed but not cured. Getting to the point where being in touch with our spiritual strength allows us to face the future with courage and intention is a worthy goal. To live each day as a gift, focusing not on the disease but on the gift of life is an important kind of healing.

As health care professionals we have the opportunity of pointing our patients to this deeper level of hope. One of the best ways of conveying it is to let them see it in the way we interact with them, in our eyes.

Tackle the Hard Questions Prior to the Visit

Some years ago I read *Thinking on Your Feet: The Art of Thinking and Speaking Under Pressure* (Wydro, 1981). It mentioned that if you are going into a difficult situation and do not know what you are going to say or do pretend you are sitting in a boat next to the dock. The dock represents the situation you have to face. In your mind, slowly paddle out into the water until you are far away from the dock. While floating on the water think through how you want to handle the situation. When your mental preparation is complete, row back to the dock and face the problem. This sounds like a gimmick, but it actually works. In life we need to take time away from our challenges to decide how to handle them.

Before some hospital visits, particularly when dealing with spiritual aspects, you may be aware that your patient is wrestling with hard questions and might address them to you. Rather than avoiding the patient's issues, row out from the dock. When possible, seek counsel from others who have had years of experience. Many physicians and other caregivers over the years have gained a wealth of helpful information dealing with the human condition, both physical and spiritual. There are not many new questions. Most challenges patients face, both spiritual and physical, are routinely seen by medical staff. Tapping the wisdom of others can add substance to your usefulness.

Network

Last, no one person should try to carry the full responsibility of spiritual care for a patient. I frequently hear, "Chaplain, I hesitate to enter a person's emotional and spiritual life for fear of opening issues I will not have time to address." In the hospital setting there is a team to work with. When issues arise there are people to call on for patient support and follow-through. The challenge is to use the team.

Within most hospitals there are chaplains, social workers, and others patients can be referred to in time of need. Outside the hospital pastors or other spiritual mentors familiar with the patient will be willing to be a spiritual resource for them. One question I often ask patients is, "Do you have a pastor or personal friend you trust with your spiritual journey that I may contact for you?"

Our responsibility is not only to personally address spiritual issues but also act as a go-between to link patients with spiritual resources they may already have in place.

SUMMARY

In this chapter twelve pieces of the spiritual care puzzle were addressed:

1. Know thyself
2. Create a safe atmosphere
3. Be aware of your surroundings
4. Identify with the patient's humanness
5. Let the patient be your teacher
6. Ask well-chosen questions
7. Mirror what you hear
8. Reevaluate a patient's spiritual status
9. Anyone can pray
10. Be a person of hope
11. Tackle the hard questions prior to the visit
12. Network

Though this list is not exhaustive it does provide a solid foundation for spiritual care. The information covered will enhance your potential as a health caregiver of the highest order.

A story is told in the Bible of several individuals who, desiring to help their sick companion, cut a hole in a roof to actually lower their friend right into the presence of Jesus. The last faces the "patient" saw before he saw Jesus were the faces of his friends circling the hole above him.

Remember that the last face the patient might see before coming in contact with his or her spiritual resources is yours.

GUIDED QUESTIONS

1. What role does crisis play in an individual's spiritual journey?
2. How can one provide a safe environment to patients?
3. How does "listening" to patients help to facilitate their spirituality?
4. How can we best frame our questions to enhance a sense of spirituality for patients?
5. How can we mirror what we hear?
6. What are some of the key points we need to remember when we pray for patients?

REFERENCES

Allender, Dan B. (1999). *The healing path*. Colorado Springs, CO: Waterbrook Press.

Kushner, Harold S. (1981). *When bad things happen to good people*. New York: Schocken Books.

Robinson, Duke (1997). *Good intentions*. New York: Warner Books.

Wydro, Kenneth (1981). *Thinking on your feet: The art of thinking and speaking under pressure*. Englewood Cliffs, NJ: Prentice-Hall.

Chapter 6

Spiritual Care of the Dying and Bereaved

Carla Gober

OBJECTIVES

1. To describe the bereavement process in regard to religious, cultural, and gender variations.
2. To discuss a multidisciplinary perspective of providing emotional, mental, and spiritual care.
3. To highlight the importance of health care professionals addressing their own physical, emotional, and spiritual needs as a condition of providing optimal care for the dying and bereaved.

INTRODUCTION

On morning rounds, the medical team stops in front of hospital room 74B. With charts open, they rehearse previous conclusions and go over lab reports, Then an odd silence develops. It is the silence that occurs when the focus changes from living to dying, from increasing the activity of saving a life to ceasing that activity altogether.

Invading this silence is the face of the little boy in 74B. He is a "near-drowning victim," but his parents do not understand the word "near" and would be distanced by the word "victim." To them, he is their son Jason, four years old. Several days ago Jason wandered into his backyard and fell into the swimming pool during the time it took his father to answer the telephone. By the time his father found him, only minutes later, Jason was unconscious. In the hospital bed, he appears to be sleeping peacefully, except for the tubes connecting him to life, and the machines recording the existence of that life. His parents, Linda and John, wait for some word that Jason will wake up, and though they fail to hear it, they continually question, watch the monitors, and imagine that they see signs of movement or wakening. In the anxiety of waiting, Linda begins to blame John for leaving the gate to the pool open and for not watching Jason. John, who already blames himself, spends less and less time in the hospital room, and more and more time in the hall and at the nurses' desk asking questions and requesting to see the physician.

There is silence during this morning's rounds because the medical team knows, and is about to acknowledge, that Jason will die. Surrounded by the most advanced medical technology and the most highly educated medical staff, all will admit that nothing more can be done to save his life. In this environment of healing, dying will take place.

Health care professionals will help determine what kind of dying this will be. Research and writing on the importance and effectiveness of bereavement care have shown the difference it makes to patient and family outcomes. In this chapter effective ways of caring for the bereaved will be discussed.

Professionals caught between living and dying often retreat to spend more time with patients who have a chance for survival. This is understandable, since saving lives is the focus of the health care professions. Many believe that once death is imminent, "nothing more can be done." This coincides with our death-denying Western culture which finds it easier to pretend there is no death than to face and treat its "sting." However, from the delivery of difficult news to the pronouncement of death and the discussions afterward, there is much more that physicians, nurses, therapists, chaplains, and other medical staff can do. What they do, or fail to do, makes a significant difference in the lives of the bereaved.

To deal with dying and death, health care professionals should redefine the goals of medical treatment to include more than saving lives. In the Bible, there are two words very closely connected, *shalem* (wholeness), and *shalom* (health/peace). Both come from the same biblical root, Sh-L-M, and illustrate its dual meaning. In this one word, health, peace, and wholeness are related. Health means more than the absence of disease; it relates to peace and the interrelatedness of the mental, spiritual, physical, emotional, social, and cultural aspects of life. The various dimensions of each person are so in-terrelated that touching one area results in touching several areas.

For example, the simple gesture of a physician asking the family if they have any questions or concerns addresses both physical and emotional needs. It may even provide opportunities for addressing spiritual needs. The various human dimensions cannot be separated from one another. In this context, helping a person physically, spiritu-ally, emotionally, and socially, whether they are living or dying, is the goal of medical treatment. Attention to health, peace, and wholeness means giving attention to the patient and his or her family.[1] It is atten-tion to the "whole person" within the "whole context."

In this chapter, this kind of care is referred to as "whole person care" and is especially beneficial to bereaved persons. Grief and mourning are complex phenomena. Grief touches every dimension of life. Although emotion is the most prominent dimension observed, there are also changes in cognitive, physical, behavioral, social, and spiritual realms.

Increasingly, medical professionals are gaining an understanding of the role of spirituality in the healing process. Classes in spiritual care have been added to medical and nursing programs as well as to educational programs for other health care professionals.

Although it is important to understand the spiritual needs of all pa-tients, this becomes especially important in death and dying situa-tions. People who have anxieties about dying identify spiritual con-cerns among their top issues. These include concerns about being forgiven by God, not reconciling with others, and dying while distant or cut off from God or a higher power (George H. Gallup Interna-tional Institute, 1997). These and other spiritual issues are often re-ferred to the chaplain. However, the various dimensions of the patient cannot always be conveniently separated along the lines of the pro-fessional disciplines. One patient tells a nurse, "If God were like you I think I would like him better." The nurse had not talked of God or of spiritual issues, yet something spiritual had been conveyed to this pa-tient. In another example, a patient asks a surgeon to pray with him before surgery to help calm his fears. This request is not surprising. In one study of cardiac surgery patients who reported on the use of prayer, 96 percent said that prayer helped them deal with the stress of surgery (Kinney, Brown, and Young-Ward, 1991). In this situation, the surgeon did not feel comfortable praying out loud, so he asked a nearby chaplain to pray, but remained in the room during the prayer. The patient thanked the surgeon for staying during the prayer, stating, "Just having you here during the prayer was helpful."

Spiritual care is a part of whole person care and can be included to some degree by every medical professional. It is an important part of a multidisciplinary approach to treating the whole person within the whole context.

DIFFICULT NEWS

In the case of Jason, the medical staff must give difficult news to Linda and John, the parents of Jason. This is generally perceived by physicians to be their role (Kayashima and Braun, 2001), but various types of difficult or bad news are also given by other members of the health care team. Delivering difficult news could include a dentist having to explain that a problem with the gums may be cancer, a physical therapist describing progressive loss of function to a cancer patient, or a chaplain admitting that she cannot explain why a good God would allow tragedy to happen. Although the responsibility for delivering difficult news may rest primarily with physicians in the hospital setting, all medical personnel are involved either in supporting physicians in this endeavor or in delivering other types of difficult news. For this reason, knowing how to deliver difficult news is important for all medical staff, and a multidisciplinary approach will promote collaborative efforts. Without this, medical team members who are faced with questions from the family about diagnosis or prognosis will not know how much to say or what kind of support to offer.

There are several areas to address when delivering difficult news in relation to dying and death. Most important to many patients and families is the content itself, including what and how much information is provided. Second is facilitation—the setting and context in which information is given. Third is the type of emotional support provided (Parker et al., 2001).

Although each person and family is different, there are optimal ways to deliver difficult news. The medical professional is not simply performing a task, but creating a memory. Words, sounds, smells, and touch all form part of that memory. As far as content is concerned, it is important to first establish what the patient and family already know and understand. This is done through asking open-ended questions. Next, information should be given in a sensitive and straight-forward manner. Many patients and families want a significant amount of information, although not necessarily all at once. This varies somewhat with age and gender, but many patients and families want more rather than less information (Jenkins, Fallowfield, and Saul, 2001). It is important for medical staff to evaluate what and how much information people want. Sometimes various members within the same family have different needs for information.

Debbie was diagnosed with lung cancer, and from the moment of diagnosis and initial prognosis, she blocked all further discussion about her illness. She said she knew she was going to die, but did not want to talk about life support or anything related to the cancer. This created differences between the information Debbie wanted and what her family wanted to know. Differences within families present a challenge for medical staff, since it is difficult to remember who wants what. However, patients and families appreciate attempts to individualize care.

When giving difficult news, space needs to be provided for questions. Giving difficult news and then leaving quickly (which can easily happen during medical rounds) can make hearing the news more difficult. Being abandoned or left alone can be isolating and frightening. Jim, who was diagnosed with pancreatic cancer, describes hearing the news: "The doctor said I had pancreatic cancer. Then she said something about three to six months, and then something else, but I was still thinking about where the pancreas was. I wasn't sure. I always get the pancreas and the liver mixed up." Since listeners often hear this kind of news in slow motion or in bits and pieces, telling it again or referring to it at a later time can be helpful.

Context is also important. Noise reduction is achieved by talking with the family in an empty room, or by simply pulling the curtain around the patient's bed. Even the *attempt* to create privacy is interpreted by many families as a caring gesture.

Whether it is a physician, nurse, or other health care professional delivering the difficult news, some type of recognition should be made of the emotions of the patient and family. One young couple remembers how a physician told them that their preterm twenty-four-week-old baby would not survive. The mother stated, "He touched our baby, and then reached out to us saying that he was sorry to have to tell us that Natasha had very little chance for survival. He didn't say much more than that, but you could tell he cared." In this scenario, this physician did three things this mother remembers. He showed care for the baby (by touching), he showed care for the parents (by touching), and he expressed a comment of emotion and care (by saying that the news was difficult to deliver).

Some would argue that patients and families would prefer competent medical practitioners to medical practitioners who are therapeutic but not competent. However, the optimal goal is not having to choose between the two. Due to overwork, lack of sleep, and constant encounters with death situations, medical professionals do not always *feel* sadness or any other emotion. One does not have to feel emotion in order to *respond* to the emotions of others. It can be a choice.

Even though difficult news may be delivered in the best possible way, the response cannot be predicted. One young woman responded violently when a physician told her that her six-year-old daughter would probably not survive the seizure that had caused her unconsciousness. The mother began screaming that it was due to the negligence of the staff and that she was going to sue the hospital. Later, this mother admitted that she felt her daughter's condition resulted from her own negligence. In trying to deal with guilt, she projected it outward onto the staff. It had nothing to do with the way the news was delivered.

On the other hand, if difficult news is delivered in less than optimal ways, the results can be devastating. Some families report bad dreams or nightmares about the way news was delivered. Others say they hear the words repeating over and over in their minds. Still others, long after the hospitalization experience, describe the uncaring attitude that accompanied delivery of the news.

Finally, responding to the emotions of others involves making sure that some type of support is available. The patient or family may have support people they want to involve, and often appreciate the support of a social worker, chaplain, or nurse after the news is given. Because this is a multidisciplinary effort, it is helpful if the one delivering the news lets other members of the medical team know what is happening and what has been said.

THE BEREAVEMENT PROCESS

Providing good bereavement care is complicated. Although medical schools, nursing schools, and other schools involved in training medical professionals now include information on bereavement care, there are still misunderstandings about behaviors and feelings surrounding death. For example, when a woman experiences a miscarriage, there is no birth certificate to mark the existence of that lost life. Sometimes mothers appear at the hospital with the remains of the miscarriage contents in a bag since most miscarriages occur outside the hospital setting or doctor's office. After being examined and checked for further bleeding they return home. There is no record that any baby existed, yet most women who miscarry feel as though they have experienced the death of their baby and experience the grief that comes with that. They are confused. If no baby actually existed, they often question if they should call themselves mothers or feel grief. Hospitals and clinics are becoming more aware of the feelings of loss these mothers experience. No official birth certificates are given, and in cases of very early gestation it is difficult to know the sex of the baby without further testing but health care professionals can encourage parents to see and name their babies. Some mothers have a sense about whether the baby was a boy or a girl and choose appropriate names. Even though medical staff may spend relatively little time with these women, they can explain the grief that may follow. They can also discuss the fact that their spouses may grieve differently because a different type of bonding occurs between men and women before the birth takes place. These are some examples of unique aspects of grief that are not often discussed in educational institutions.

There are several types of losses and multiple theories about how people progress through grief. Mourning follows the loss of anything meaningful or anyone connected in meaningful ways. No particular type of loss can be categorized as insignificant if it is significant to those connected with it. Even the death of a bird or animal can be significant, and can elicit a grief response.

The professional literature uses several terms to describe the process of bereavement. According to Corr (2000), *grief* generally refers to the subjective reaction to a loss while *bereavement* refers to the objective state of having suffered a loss. *Mourning* refers to "the conscious and unconscious intrapsychic processes, together with the cultural, public, or interpersonal efforts, that are involved in attempts to cope with loss and grief" (Corr, 2000, p. 22). Mourning is a long-term process that involves reorientation of the relationship to the deceased, an altered sense of self, and a changed view of the external world.

Theorists have described grief in terms of stages, phases, and tasks. In her book, *On Death and Dying,* Elisabeth Kübler-Ross (1969) identifies five *stages* of grief reactions: denial, anger, bargaining, depression, and acceptance/decathexis. Since her study involved those who were dying and their reactions to their own impending deaths, it stands to reason that grief reactions over the death of a loved one (the bereaved) might be different. John Bowlby (1980) identifies three *phases:* the urge to recover the lost object, disorganization and despair, and reorganization. Colin Murray Parkes (2001) later modified this (with modifications agreed to by Bowlby) to four phases: shock and numbness, searching and yearning, disorganization and despair, and reorganization. Rando (1993) discusses mourning in terms of reactions and identifies them as avoidance, confrontation, and reestablishment. Another theorist, William Worden (1991), describes a model of mourning in terms of *tasks.* All of these theories, whether based on stages, phases, or tasks, illustrate that the mourning process involves extended time and a variety of responses. Rather than reaching a positive end to grief (such as *acceptance* in the stages of Kübler-Ross, 1969), some theorists suggest that there really is no end to the mourning process; rather it is a process of readjustment that lasts a lifetime.

Although there may be no one specific order in which the bereaved adjust to loss, the four phases as identified by Bowlby (1980) and Parkes (2001) are used for this chapter. The first phase involves aspects of shock, disbelief, and numbness. This is the phase that families experience while in the hospital setting. Shock acts as a protective mechanism against the full effects of the loss. During this time, new information is difficult to assimilate and denial temporarily protects from some of the pain.

Lyle is seventy-five years old and stares out the window after hearing the news that his wife died in surgery. He responds to the surgeon, "Are you absolutely sure? I can't live without her, you know." In another example, Maria, a fifty-five-year-old woman, sits beside the bed of her husband Juan, who has gastrointestinal bleeding and hepatic failure. She knows her husband will die, but does not want him to know that she knows. Juan tells the staff that he knows of his impending death, but does not want his wife to know because it will "cause her pain." She sits beside his bed and they talk of other things. In a third example, David is a young father who calls the physician six weeks after his baby dies. He states, "I know you told us what caused the death of Amber, but could you tell us again? We can't remember some of what you said and we have a lot of questions." In a fourth example, a middle-aged couple is in a car accident. The wife, Jenny, dies in the emergency room, and the husband, Tom, is in the same hospital for observation and traction. He is not able to go to the funeral, so the family has decided to have the funeral without him. All of these are examples of difficulties that can surround shock and numbness. Facts are given to patients and families during this time and many decisions have to be made. All of this is especially difficult when the body is in a slowed down, protective mode.

Health care professionals may find it difficult to know which responsibilities belong to whom in these contexts. In some health care facilities, whether clinic or hospital, these roles are clearly defined and specific members of the medical team are responsible for grief care. However, the most optimal grief care comes from a multidisciplinary approach. In the case of Lyle, whose wife died in surgery, it is the surgeon who gives him the news about the death of his wife. The reality is that the surgeon also has several other cases. The other part of that reality is that this gentleman is at high risk for health problems within the next year as a result of the unbearable loneliness this loss may create in his life. How the surgeon responds to this dilemma is not a matter of time as much as choice. In the few minutes the surgeon has with this man, care can be shown along with giving the facts, and provision can be made for further support. Making provision for further support involves notifying the nurse of what is taking place and providing for chaplain referral if that is desired. The surgeon does not have to *provide* the grief care, but has the choice of whether to open up other avenues of support.

In the case of Maria and Juan, any member of the health care team can encourage them to talk with each other, and can even facilitate that by asking a question in the presence of both of them. If they need someone to help facilitate further discussion, referral can be made. Initiating discussion between them can take place during a treatment, the giving of medications, or during rounds.

In the case of David, the young father of Amber, if the clinic personnel understand grief, they will recognize that this is very common. Parents are initially in shock and cannot take in all the information they are given. Very often they will ask the same questions weeks later as the shock and numbness begin to fade. Health care professionals should not only tolerate this, but also expect and provide for it. Questions (sometimes the same questions) surface weeks later, and therapists, clinic personnel, nurses, and physicians can promote bereavement care by planning ways to incorporate these questions into continuing care.

In the case of Tom, who was unable to attend his wife's funeral, the nurse discovered that he wanted to see and say good-bye to his deceased wife, since the last thing he remembered was her crying out for him to help her. Initially, the physician, nurse, and chaplain worked together to provide a way for this to happen. A slanted mirror was placed in such a way as to enable Tom to see her body without jeopardizing his traction. After talking to his daughter it was discovered that Jenny's body had already been transported to the crematorium. At the request of the family, the nurse called the crematorium and requested return of the body; the family decided to wait six weeks to have the funeral, and the physician discharged Tom temporarily to attend the service. Altogether, this took about twenty minutes of time from the health care team, but it made a very significant difference for Tom.

Medical staff can do several things to help during this time of shock and numbness. Facts regarding prognosis, dying, and cause of death need to be repeated at the time and later as questions arise. Families need to be encouraged to see and say good-bye to their loved ones, whether the loss is a miscarriage or the death of a longtime companion. Even after bodies have been transported to the morgue, viewing is often still possible. In the case of newborn deformity, parents can decide how much of the baby they want to view. If a baby has anencephaly (missing part or all of the brain), small hats can be placed on the head of the baby to ease the viewing process. Parents can choose whether or not to remove the hat or blanket that covers the deformity. Many families are not aware of this. One father had a baby with facial disfigurement (cycloptic). He chose to view the baby, while the mother chose not to. When first seeing his baby son, the father stated, "He has my hands, doesn't he?" When viewing the face he responded, "Hmmm. He's not a monster; he's just deformed." Within the next two years, this father wanted to have more children. His wife refused. In her mind, her body had produced a monster, and this perception of failure prevented her from wanting more children. Choosing not to see and hold her baby had implications for the future. This can also be true for families and loved ones who may have been at the bedside during illness; sometimes being there at the time of death can be very important.

Children's involvement in the dying process should be handled carefully but realistically. Kastenbaum (2000, p. 19) suggests that it is easy for us to think of childhood as "the kingdom where nobody dies," but as much as we would like to protect children from death, it is neither possible nor advisable. Although children cannot be protected from death, it is important to prepare them for a death that is inevitable or has occurred, and to know how to support them in ways that are appropriate for their age. According to Fry (2000), children do better with dying situations when they are given concrete information about the disease beforehand. Evasive answers only cause children to make up their own stories about what they perceive to be causing anxiety in the family. Even therapies and treatment can be simply explained in concrete terms. If play therapists are a part of the medical team, they can help prepare children through creative play, painting, crafts, and rituals.

The particular age at which all children can view a deceased body or attend a funeral depends on each child. After describing the disease process and giving concrete information about what the child can expect to see, they need to be given a choice about how to participate. This can happen as soon as they are developmentally able to understand and make that choice. After hearing the description of what he would look like, six-year-old Kayla was given the choice to see her deceased newborn brother. She decided that she would and stretched out her arms to receive him. Helping her hold her brother, her mother talked with her about his hands, fingers, and toes. Fearing that Kayla would cry, her mother was shocked when Kayla looked up at her and responded excitedly, "He looks just like my doll! I want to keep him for a while." In this way, children and adolescents enter into the grieving process instead of being isolated and separated from the family. If they are not given the opportunity to understand the reason for the tears and sadness, they may assume blame for it themselves.

This issue becomes especially important with the death of a parent. For children, the early loss of a parent creates particular challenges that extend into adulthood. Because this is one of the most difficult types of loss for a child, specific care needs to be taken to help children cope in the initial phases of grief.

Medical staff cannot possibly understand all the dynamics of a particular family during this time. Often there have been previous unresolved losses, conflicted relationships, unspoken resentments, and feelings of guilt. All of this is augmented during a time of grief and mourning. The health care team is not responsible for this, or even for understanding all of it. However, by working together, the team can facilitate healthy grieving.

When families are saying good-bye to their loved ones, privacy is needed. Screens can be placed around families if they are in environments where complete privacy is not possible (as is often the case in neonatal intensive care units). During this process, door cards can be placed on the screen or door of the room to alert the health care team about what is taking place. If the rest of the team is not aware, their actions may not be conducive to the grieving process. One housekeeper recalls, "I was humming and singing to myself when I went into the room of one mom. I saw her with her baby and told her how happy I was for her. Suddenly I realized she was crying as she held him. Then I saw that he wasn't breathing. I didn't know what to say then." This type of thing can be avoided if the health care team is alerted in some way.

The second phase of bereavement involves searching, yearning, and attempts to recover the lost object or person. During this phase many people feel that they are "going crazy." Bereaved mothers may experience aching arms, some adults experience pains in the chest that simulate angina, and others experience weight loss or gain, various body aches, and problems sleeping at night. By this time, families and loved ones generally do not have direct contact with the hospital setting, but it is important for medical staff, especially in treatment, office, or clinic settings to recognize these symptoms. For example, bereaved mothers who have refused to take medication to dry up their milk may return to the physician during this time for problems of engorgement. This is a physical problem, but it is also a problem relating to the mourning process. Although all pains and aches should be assessed as potential health problems, it is important to assess whether the person who experiences them has had a recent major loss. This part of the bereavement process is eased somewhat if families and loved ones have been encouraged early on by medical staff to attend support groups or seek counseling.

Depression, disorganization, and disorientation characterize the third phase of the bereavement process. Very often people withdraw from others, resort to substance abuse, and experience hesitancy in seeking help. Sometimes they show up in medical offices or clinic settings with complaints of depression, loss of energy, and difficulty performing work and home tasks. Again, it is easy for the medical professional to fail to correctly assess the reason for these symptoms, which are often especially pronounced on the one-year anniversary of the death.

Finally, resolution marks the fourth phase of the bereavement process. Although this may seem to be an easy phase, the bereaved often feel guilty about feeling good again. By discussing this before it takes place, the bereaved are not caught off guard by the guilt that often accompanies it. Instead, they feel permission to experience joy again.

Although medical staff, especially within the hospital setting, will see more of the first phase of bereavement than the following three phases, understanding the entire grief process will enable staff to know how to talk with families about what they can expect.

The most effective bereavement care occurs when there is an organized multidisciplinary approach to providing it. In some hospitals, a checklist is attached to the chart to provide a place for various health care personnel to chart bereavement care. This includes visits by the physician, chaplain referral, social worker referral, opportunities for viewing the deceased, memory items (photos, handprints or footprints in the case of babies, and cards), funeral arrangements, grief process, and other issues related to bereavement care. By having one designated place to record grief care, various members of the team are able to collaborate with one another, and a more unified approach is possible.

RELIGIOUS, SPIRITUAL, AND CULTURAL ISSUES

When a person is dying or loved ones are grieving a death, often questions arise about spiritual and religious issues. Questions such as, "Why me? Why now? Why this?" are voiced. Many have questions about healing miracles, what happens after death, and about God's presence or absence in the process of dying. These issues can be referred to a pastor or chaplain. Sometimes patients or family members ask questions of the ones from whom they desire responses. They may have grown close to a specific physician, nurse, respiratory therapist, or other member of the health care team, and trust their questions with that person. Sometimes questions come out at odd times or in what seem to be unusual ways. Ben had severe congestive heart failure, could hardly move in bed, and was unable to walk. When the physician was making morning rounds, Ben whispered, "Doc, I want to die." Since he had such difficulty breathing, that sentence required several intervening breaths. In trying to think of ways to help Ben be hopeful, the physician ended up saying nothing. Ben filled the silence, "I'm ready to go, and God knows that." Several referrals were made and finally Ben told a chaplain, "You all are making a huge effort to make me want to live, but I just wanted the doc to know that I'm ready to go." After Ben was discharged, he stopped taking all medications and died in his sleep. His desire had been a simple one. He wanted his physician and others to know that he was ready to die.

Religious and spiritual issues are often uncomfortable for health care professionals, for various reasons. Some feel that spiritual concerns are outside the realm of professional practice. Others have personal conflicts in this area and feel incapable of dealing with them. Still others fear saying the wrong thing, or not knowing what to say, especially in cases in which religious views differ from their own. Certainly, it is always appropriate to offer chaplain referral. In many cases people do not want answers as much as they want to express their questions and feelings. Health care professionals can give what time they have, and then provide other options. Patients and families understand time constraints. What they are less able to understand is avoidance and abandonment.

Beliefs about healing and mourning vary with religious and cultural groups. One elderly woman sat in a chair beside the bed of her dying husband. The respiratory therapist came in to give a treatment and the wife whispered to the therapist, "I am at peace. I know my husband will not be reborn as a lower form of animal." The therapist listened and nodded, unsure of how to respond to this Buddhist woman. Various religions teach that death is not the complete end of the human spirit, and have rituals and funeral practices surrounding these beliefs. Although others may not believe in an afterlife, they still struggle to make sense of suffering and death. Medical professionals can help in this area by including questions about religious preference in their assessments, and by continuing to assess spiritual needs throughout the dying process.

Some medical professionals wonder if it is appropriate to "share the gospel" with patients and families. This is a sensitive area. In one situation, a medical professional felt it was his duty to "share the gospel" with every patient who was dying. In his mind this meant conversion to Christianity. Even though one patient refused, this professional proceeded. This goes against patient rights and is inappropriate. On the other hand, often in life-threatening situations, people want a sense of connection or peace with God. Some look back on their lives with guilt and would rather talk with a medical professional than a religious representative. Medical professionals need to check hospital policy to find out what is encouraged within their particular setting. If it is within hospital policy, medical professionals can best deal with these issues by sensitively investigating the need as well as how to address that need without forcing a particular endpoint. Sometimes a patient or family wants prayer, scripture reading, or someone to listen. In other cases, patients and families have particular questions for which they want answers. In cases where questions occur about forgiveness or acceptance by God, the reading of scripture can be as helpful as an explanation. The most important thing is for the medical professional to assess the need. A good example of this is found in the New Testament. When encountering blind men, Jesus asked them, "What do you want me to do for you?" The answer to this question seems obvious. Blind men call out to the one who is reputed to heal blindness. However, Jesus seems to assume nothing. This is not to suggest that he would have responded in any way they wanted. Rather, before doing something to or for them, he asked them what they wanted. Rightly assessing a need is an important step in providing spiritual care.

Sometimes patients and families want something the medical professional cannot give, such as time, answers, specific interventions, or healing. During a physical therapy treatment, a woman with metastatic breast cancer asked the therapist why God would "allow this to happen." The therapist was not a religious person and did not feel comfortable talking about religious issues. Rather than ignore the question, she let the woman know that she did not feel competent in this area and would call the chaplain if the woman would like that. In this case, the chaplain was called and the conversation continued within that context. The need was not left unattended.

In the case of a chaplain referral, questions arise about how much information should be shared with the rest of the medical team since conversations may be private in nature. It is helpful if chaplains chart short summaries of their visits, especially when specific issues could impact care. One woman explained to the chaplain that she was refusing treatment because she thought her ovarian cancer was a judgment from God for an affair she had. This type of information directly affects treatment and is important for the rest of the medical team to know. At the very least, the chaplain can stamp the chart or mark the daily activity sheet to show that spiritual care is being provided. When staff meet as a multidisciplinary team to plan patient care, chaplain and social worker involvement is important.

Monica McGoldrick (1989) discusses the importance of understanding a family's cultural practices surrounding death, rituals, and the afterlife. Failing to understand these practices may inhibit grief care or a family's ability to progress through the mourning process. One six-year-old female patient lay unconscious from what the parents declared to be a fall from a tree. The medical staff noticed small round sores on her back that appeared to be from cigarette burns. Child abuse was suspected. It was not until appropriate translators could be found that the cultural practice of "coining" was understood to have caused the sores. Turning a coin on its edge, a family member would turn it in circular motion, creating a perfectly round mark on the skin for the purpose of "letting the pain out." With better understanding of this family's cultural practices, the medical staff was better able to discuss "brain death" and help the family see that their daughter was not in pain, even though she would not get better. The same discussion would not have been possible if the parents had continued to be suspected of child abuse.

If the family or loved ones are not encouraged to maintain their cultural traditions, the mourning process can be hindered. One intensive care nurse complained that "too many family members are in the room and they are making too much noise." The patient was Hispanic. Upon his death, there were more than ten family members present. The patient's brother was bumping his head on the wall as an expression of grief. When asked if she thought any of them were in danger of hurting themselves, the nurse felt that they were not. The patient was in a room by himself, so no other patients were being disturbed. The nurse realized that she was uncomfortable with the way this family was expressing grief, not because it was harmful to the family or other patients, but because it seemed peculiar to her. Realizing that this expression was helpful to the family and loved ones, she closed the door and allowed them privacy to grieve.

Although it is impossible to know and understand all religious and cultural traditions, it is important for medical professionals to have a cursory knowledge of those that are most frequently encountered and to be aware of resources that can help.

Gender Differences

Across cultures, there tend to be different expectations about mourning for women and men. This is not to say that all women or all men grieve according to gender expectations or that all men or women of a given culture grieve similarly; some differences between women and men can be expected. Following the death of a stillborn baby, Thomas and Striegel (1995) reported the tendency of men to contain their grief in an attempt to care for their wives. They concluded that while the women in their study grieved for the loss of their babies, the men tended to grieve for their wives.

Studies on widows and widowers also show differences. Parkes (2001) suggests that widowed women show more overt signs of distress from initial grief while widowed men show more long-lasting effects. Parkes attributes this difference to the tendency of men to contain rather than express their grief. It may also represent the tendency to grieve differently. Many men choose anger as a vehicle for expressing grief, while women often choose sadness. However, according to Martin and Doka (2000), these differences may relate more to patterns of grieving and gender role socialization than to innate gender-related expressions of grief.

In cultures in which acceptable grief is defined to be expression of sadness through tears and communal sharing, expression of grief as aggression, anger, or withdrawal may not be as acceptable. Men and women should be encouraged to grieve the way they each need to grieve. Medical professionals should acknowledge all forms of grief and help families and loved ones share in that grief.

William Worden (1996) suggests four tasks for the grieving individual, and Walsh and McGoldrick (1988) broaden them to represent the experiences that are necessary for a family or social system. The four tasks are: shared acknowledgment of the reality of death, shared experience of the pain of grief, reorganization of the family system, and redirection of relationships and goals. Doka (1993) adds one more task to represent the spiritual dimension: reconstruction of faith and philosophical systems that have been challenged by loss. For all of these to occur, differences in expression of grief must be understood. If family and loved ones are not forewarned of this possibility, they may separate from one another as their expectations for expressions of grief from others are not met.

A mother complained to the physician that her husband did not feel sad about the loss of their child. The father was stunned. He replied, "I feel so sad that I can hardly even function, but I'm trying to be strong. Somebody needs to hold this family together." Often, one person does not realize that another person is uncomfortable with the way he or she expresses grief. One of the greatest gifts the medical professional can give is helping families and loved ones realize that their experiences and expressions of grief may differ over time, and this is normal. A statement like this can be made by anyone on the health care team, and will enable families and loved ones to interpret one another more appropriately by understanding and expecting these differences ahead of time. During a return visit to the hospital, one woman confided to the nursing staff, "You all told us that we might grieve differently, and you were right. I keep thinking of that when I see my husband work all the time and then sit quietly for hours in front of the TV without really watching it."

Abnormal Grief

One of the purposes of providing effective grief care is to decrease the risk for abnormal grief. Elliott Rosen (1998, p. 111) defines abnormal grief as "too little grieving immediately after a death or too much grieving long afterward." Many things contribute to people grieving too little or too much, some of which can be avoided and some of which cannot. The early loss of a parent can predispose adults to abnormal grief, as can circumstances surrounding the death, such as not viewing the body (due to major burns or body mutilation), or refusal by loved ones to allow specific people to view the body, as is often the case with children. Ambiguous loss, or loss that is unclear or indeterminate (such as happens with drowning, airplane crashes, abduction, and war) (Boss, 1999) often contributes to problems in grieving. Helping patients and families effectively grieve during the initial phases of grief will decrease the risk for abnormal grief.

FOLLOW-UP CARE

In working with the bereaved, follow-up care is needed. In some medical settings, chaplains, social workers, or hospice workers provide follow-up care. In other settings, volunteers do phone follow-up to assess family functioning and offer support. Again, the most effective type of follow-up is multidisciplinary. Some neonatologists plan for follow-up phone calls to answer questions they know parents will have around issues such as the cause of death, genetic testing, and future pregnancy. Hospital chaplains are often asked to perform the funeral services. Nurses frequently send condolence cards. One family told the pediatric medical staff that the card they received from the staff meant more to them than any other card they received. Sometimes the staff does not realize how important they become to families in the joint struggle against impending death, and the later struggle to deal with the grief that results from that death.

Often physicians, nurses, chaplains, and other medical staff will attend the funerals of patients with whom they have worked. By doing this, they offer empathy to the families and bring closure for themselves as well. Jason's story is particularly relevant here. As mentioned at the beginning of this chapter, Jason was four years old and was found by his father in the swimming pool. Eventually, life support was discontinued and plans for burial were made. The medical staff was invited to the funeral. A physician, social worker, and several nurses attended, and a priest officiated at the graveside. After a few words to the family, the priest took off his vestments and in street clothes walked to the back of the crowd. As the crowd watched in silence, the priest took the arm of the physician and pulled him forward to stand with him and the parents beside the small white casket. Other family members and medical staff stood close by. It seemed to be an admission by all that in the struggle for life, all had done what they could, including God, medicine, and human love.

This story is ideal and certainly does not represent the way of all death scenarios. It is impossible for staff to attend all funerals, or even to feel close to all families that experience a loss. It is used simply to illustrate times when medical professionals find it helpful to attend funerals, for the sake of the families as well as themselves.

THE MEDICAL PROFESSIONAL

When providing whole person care to people who are dying or bereaved, medical professionals encounter several challenges. Often they have their own unresolved personal issues related to loss and death. A young nurse may find it extremely difficult to work with grief situations in labor and delivery since she experienced the death of her own baby. A respiratory therapist may find it difficult to give treatments to lung cancer patients since his father died of lung cancer. An emergency room physician called to a SIDS (sudden infant death syndrome) death only to discover that the baby is his own will continue to struggle with grief situations in the emergency room. Recently treated for breast cancer, a female physician may struggle when taking care of dying female patients.

For a variety of reasons, providing grief care is challenging for the health care professional. This should not be ignored. When there is personal unresolved grief, it can impede care for others. The opposite can also be true. Continuing to provide grief care can augment personal unresolved losses.

Two suggestions may help health care professionals dealing with their own grief. First, medical professionals need to be aware of their own losses and how these impact current personal functioning. If possible, some situations should be avoided, and time off can provide space for healing. If medical professionals are oblivious to their own woundedness, they may become bitter, edgy, isolated, or difficult.

Second, medical professionals who work around death and dying need a plan for helping one another cope with crisis situations. For instance, in one emergency room, a crisis intervention plan was developed. On one occasion after an attempted resuscitation, the team was invited to attend a short time of debriefing. The staff thought they were too busy and did not need it. However, once they gathered, they talked about how much they were affected by several aspects of the experience. For one medical professional, the five-year-old they attempted to resuscitate reminded him of his own five-year-old son. For another, trying to comfort the mother who kept screaming for her son to live was difficult. It raised questions about whether family members should be allowed in the room. Others talked of experiencing the failure to save a life. All of them expressed appreciation for the opportunity to thank each team member for doing all that could be done.

Burnout, depression, and job dissatisfaction can result when there is no plan of care for the medical professional. Optimal bereavement care is a response to the "whole person" within the "whole context." Part of that context is the world of the medical professional.

Finally, in order for the medical professional to provide spiritual care, personal spiritual needs must be addressed. Henri Nouwen (1990) uses the term "wounded healer." He suggests that out of his or her own woundedness, the healer reaches out to others. Part of this includes acknowledging personal needs for forgiveness and reconciliation, simple needs for sleep and support, the challenge of personal limitations, and the inability to save all lives. At times, spiritual care comes from the patient and family in allowing the medical professional to share in a story that has the capacity to change life, even the life of the health care professional.

GUIDED QUESTIONS

1. What are the three areas that one should address in communicating bad news?
2. What are the four stages of the bereavement process? What should one pay attention to during various stages of the bereavement process?
3. What are some of the spiritual issues one should be aware of?
4. What are some basic gender differences in grief?
5. Define abnormal grief.
6. What factors have the potential to cause abnormal grief?

NOTE

1. The definition of "family" used in this chapter is taken from Pauline Boss (1999) in her book, *Ambiguous Loss,* p. 4. She writes: "By family I mean that intimate group of people whom we can count on over time for comfort, care, nurturance, support, sustenance, and emotional closeness. Family can be people with whom we grew up—called the family of origin—or it can be people we select in adulthood—called the family of choice. The latter may include biological or nonbiological offspring or no offspring at all. . . .This view of family stresses the criterion of being present—psychologically and physically—even more than that of being biologically related."

REFERENCES

Boss, P. (1999). *Ambiguous Loss. Learning to Live with Unresolved Grief.* Cambridge: Harvard University Press.

Bowlby, J. (1980). *Attachment and Loss: Volume 3, Loss, Sadness and Depression.* New York: Basic Books.

Corr, C.A. (2000). What Do We Know About Grieving Children and Adolescents? In *Living with Grief: Children, Adolescents, and Loss,* K. Doka (Ed.) (pp. 21-34). Washington, DC: Hospice Foundation of America: Brunner/Mazel.

Doka, K.J. and Morgan, J. (1993). *Death and Spirituality.* Amityville, NY: Baywood.

Fry, V.L. (2000). Part of Me Died Too: Creative Strategies for Grieving Children and Adolescents. In *Living with Grief: Children, Adolescents, and Loss,* K. Doka (Ed.) (pp. 125-138). Washington, DC: Hospice Foundation of America: Brunner/Mazel.

George H. Gallup International Institute (1997). *Spiritual Beliefs and the Dying Process: A Report on a National Survey.* Princeton, NJ: Princeton Religious Research Center.

Jenkins, V., Fallowfield, L., and Saul, J. (2001). Information Needs of Patients with Cancer: Results from a Large Study in UK Cancer Centres. *British Journal of Cancer,* 84(1):48-51.

Kastenbaum, R. (2000). The Kingdom Where Nobody Dies. In *Living with Grief: Children, Adolescents, and Loss,* K. Doka (Ed.) (pp. 5-20). Washington, DC: Hospice Foundation of America: Brunner/Mazel.

Kayashima, R. and Braun, K.L. (2001). Barriers to Good End of Life Care: A Physician Survey. *Hawaii Medical Journal,* 60(2):40-44.

Kinney, S.T.L., Brown, K.D., and Young-Ward, L. (1991). Health Locus of Control and Helpfulness of Prayer. *Heart and Lung,* 20(1):60-65.

Kübler-Ross, E. (1969). *On Death and Dying.* London: Tavistock.

Martin, T. and Doka, K. (2000). *Men Don't Cry. . .Women Do. Transcending Gender Stereotypes of Grief.* Philadelphia: Brunner/Mazel.

Matthews, D.A., Larson, D.B., and Barry, C.P. (1993). *The Faith Factor: An Annotated Bibliography of Clinical Research on Spiritual Subjects.* Radnor, PA: John Templeton Foundation.

McGoldrick, M. (1989). Ethnicity and the Family Life Cycle. In *The Changing Family Life Cycle: A Framework for Family Therapy,* B. Carter and M. McGoldrick (Eds.) (pp. 69-90). Boston: Allyn & Bacon.

Nouwen, H. (1990). *The Wounded Healer: Ministry in Contemporary Society.* New York: Image Books.

Parker, P.A., Baile, W.F., deMoor, C., Lenzi, R., Kudelka, A.P., and Cohen, L. (2001). Breaking Bad News About Cancer: Patients' Preferences for Communication. *Journal of Clinical Oncology,* 19(7):2049-2056.

Parkes, C.M. (2001). *Bereavement: Studies of Grief in Adult Life,* Third Edition. Philadelphia: Taylor and Francis Group.

Rando, T. (1993). *Treatment of Complicated Mourning.* Champaign, IL: Research Press.

Rosen, E. J. (1998). *Families Facing Death: A Guide for Healthcare Professionals and Volunteers.* San Francisco: Jossey-Bass Publishers.

Thomas, V. and Striegel, P. (1995). Stress and Grief of a Perinatal Loss: Integrating Qualitative and Quantitative Methods. *Omega,* 30(4): 299-311.

Walsh, F. and McGoldrick, M. (1988). Loss and the Family Life Cycle. *Family Transitions: Continuity and Change over the Life Cycle.* In C.J. Falicov (Ed.) (pp. 311-336). New York: Guilford Press.

Worden, J.W. (1991). *Grief Counseling and Grief Therapy,* Second Edition. New York: Springer.

Worden, J.W. (1996). *Children and Grief: When a Parent Dies.* New York: Guilford.

Chapter 7

Health, Wholeness, and Diversity: Intercultural Engagement in Health Care

Johnny Ramírez-Johnson

OBJECTIVES

1. To recognize diversity as an essential dimension of wholeness.
2. To discuss problems of availability and quality of health care for minorities.
3. To reflect on the role culture plays in expectations for and understanding of health.
4. To show a need for greater awareness of the effects cultural assumptions have on health care.
5. To reflect on the need to move away from personal comfort zones in order to minister to people from other cultural and religious backgrounds.

INTRODUCTION

This is written from a Western perspective, seeking universal humanistic principles grounded in the Christian tradition. The principle of "loving your neighbor as yourself" (Lev 19:18 and Matt 22:39, NIV) is found in the Bible, which is the central document of Christianity, as well as the injunction: "Do to others as you would have them do to you" (Lk 6:31, NIV). From a humanistic viewpoint, a point of departure for this chapter is found in the World Health Organization's (WHO) definition of health. This dual ideological tradition has been at the center of Western philosophy. It has permeated social, economic, political, and health institutions.

WHO's definition of health has universal appeal. "Health is a state of complete physical, mental and social well-being and not merely the absence of disease or infirmity" (WHO, 1948: Preamble). This definition of health as a "state" of being complete fits perfectly with the central objective of this book, the promotion of wholeness. Being complete, or the state of being complete, covers physical, mental, and social well-being of each individual with his or her uniqueness. Thus the idea of being complete or whole is a philosophical concept that assigns intrinsic value to each individual, and in so doing, advances diversity.

Although all humans have a physical side manifested in their bodily functions and expressions, all bodies are by definition unique. Diversity is clearly implied as a central attribute of any statement that describes the human body. It is an axiom that no two people are alike, either genetically, physically, or mentally.

Any effort at bettering social well-being also calls for acknowledgment of diversity. Social dimensions of all human enterprise demonstrate the diversity of the human experience. Humans seek similar aims, but in an astounding variety of ways. The preamble to the WHO constitution states, "The enjoyment of the highest attainable standard of health is one of the fundamental rights of every human being without distinction of race, religion, political belief, economic or social condition" (1948).

This aim goes along with the concept of the pursuit of happiness which is a part of the preamble to the Declaration of Independence. "We hold these truths to be self-evident, that all men are created equal, that they are endowed by their Creator with certain unalienable Rights, that among these are Life, Liberty and the pursuit of Happiness."

Many Americans naturally assume that everyone should experience a state of complete well-being. Health, as understood by the WHO, is as American as apple pie. All humans, and thus all patients, deserve equal access to well-being regardless of their race or social status. In other words, because of diversity all humans deserve wholeness, the state of being complete.

The goal of this chapter is to create greater awareness of the complexity and challenges of addressing the issue of diversity particularly within the context of health care. The American culture is the context for the exploration of the importance of cultural diversity and the need for self-awareness. Diversity in America, religion and racial discrimination, discrimination in our health care system, and three case studies will be discussed.

DIVERSITY IN AMERICA

Because humans are diverse all human endeavors benefit from perspectives that accommodate this variety of views. Patients represent all possible human populations and groups. Health care providers are also diverse. They speak a variety of languages and experience a wide spectrum of views on life, just like their patients. Therefore, issues of diversity exist in each health care institution. Commenting on the United States of America, President John F. Kennedy (1964) stated in his book, *A Nation of Immigrants,* "The three ships which discovered America sailed under a Spanish flag, were commanded by an Italian sea captain, and included in their crew an Englishman, an Irishman, a Jew and a Negro" (p. 10). From the very beginning of the American experience until the twenty-first century, America has always been defined by diversity.

A census is conducted every decade by the U.S. Department of Commerce. The latest census (2000), reported several interesting trends (see Table 7.1). Hispanics are now the largest minority group in the United States, and blacks occupy second place (12.5 percent and 12.1 percent, respectively). The nation is growing at an exponential rate, with most of the growth among minority groups. The Asian population, while representing a small minority (3.6 percent), continues to grow. The white population, although still the majority group, is not growing as fast as other groups. Population trends indicate that in a matter of decades there will be no majority group representing over 50 percent of the population.

Racial and ethnic diversity combined with diversity of household arrangements—more single mothers, more households without children, and more elderly people living alone—indicate that America is becoming older, more lonely, and more racially diverse. These changes are neither good nor bad, but simply a sign of the socioeconomic realities of affluence and development.

Language diversity in America is coupled with religious and cultural diversity. More Americans are born abroad today than any time

TABLE 7.1. Population by Race and Hispanic or Latino Origin, for All Ages, for the United States: 2000

Population groups including all ages	Totals by groups	Percent
Total U.S. population	281,421,906	100.00
Hispanic or Latino (of any race)	35,305,818	12.50
White	194,552,774	69.10
Black or African American	33,947,837	12.10
American Indian and Alaska Native	2,068,883	0.70
Asian	10,123,169	3.60
Native Hawaiian and Other Pacific Islander	353,509	0.10
Some other race	467,770	0.20
Two or more races	4,602,146	1.60

Source: U.S. Census Bureau, Internet release date April 2, 2001, <www.census.gov>.

since census data have been collected. More people speak more than one language today than ten years ago. From the perspective of health, diversity continues to play a significant role. Many issues are involved such as access to health care, availability of services, health insurance, education, socioeconomic status, and health practices. Culture also has an impact on health status.[1]

Americans are ambivalent about diversity, sometimes favoring it (when the economy is on an upward trend) and sometimes disliking it (when the economy is down).[2] The trend between 1993 and 2001 in The Gallup Poll (2003) illustrates this. When things were going well and the economy was growing, more Americans believed diversity mostly improved American culture, but in 2001 when the economy got tighter the majority felt that diversity mostly threatened American culture (see Table 7.2).

TABLE 7.2. Americans' Attitudes Toward Cultural Diversity

	Mostly improve	Mostly threaten	Both (vol.)	Neither (vol.)	No opinion
July 9-11, 1993	45	38	4	5	8
March 26-28, 2001	35	55	3	3	4

Source: The Gallup Organization, 2003

The worst manifestations of American intolerance and open violence against non-European and nonwhite members of society were in the past. Slavery was eliminated with the Emancipation Proclamation issued by President Abraham Lincoln on January 1, 1863. This edict freed the slaves in the Confederate states, and the union's victory in the Civil War ensured that their freedom would be carried out. The civil liberties of all Americans regardless of gender, race, ethnicity, and religious or political affiliation were secured by President Lyndon B. Johnson's Civil Rights Act legislation of 1964. But the philosophical culprit of racism—undermining, belittling, and otherwise abhorring one group while preferring another solely because of race, ethnicity, or culture is a matter of ideology and cannot be legislated away.

Christianity and Racial Discrimination

Discrimination based on social status, religious beliefs, physical appearance, or national identity is a universal reality. It is rooted in our inability to step beyond our comfort zone and recognize validity of others who differ from us. In America, this tendency to discriminate is mostly based on physical appearances or race.

Discrimination based on racial factors means that regardless of religious beliefs, socioeconomic status, national identity, or any other factor, an individual is classified strictly by his or her skin color and physical features. Two well-known systems using this racial ideology were American Jim Crow laws and South African apartheid. Both historical institutions are in disrepute, rejected by the nations that gave them birth; but they are still very much present in people's psyches, and many argue that they still affect social institutions, including health care.

In 1684 Francois Bernier proposed the concept of organizing humans by their phenotype (physical characteristics). (For a full discussion of the development of racism as a European ideology see: Kelsey, 1965; Jordan, 1968; Mosse, 1978; Staum, 2000.) In the 1730s Carolus Linnaeus further developed the incipient ideology that set up a conceptual framework for ranking humans into a hierarchical order, later known as "a chain of being," principally based on human phenotype (Staum, 2000).

Many others advanced the notion that humans can be placed in such qualitative hierarchical orders and a so-called "chain of being" became more and more accepted as a popular ideology (Staum, 2000). Among the principal philosophers and humanists who promoted and developed this racist ideology are: David Hume (1748); Johann Friedrich Blumenbach (1775); Johann Kaspar Lavater (1781); Christian Meiners (1785); Peter Camper (1792); Franz Joseph Gall (1796); and Charles White (1799). The first to suggest that intermarriage would harm civilization by degeneration of the white race was Mieners (Roberts, 1995).

Several other ideologies after Meiners paved the way to modern racism. Three main tracts were arguably the most influential in America: Robert Knox, *Races of Men* (1850); Carl Gustav Carus, *Symbolism of the Human Form* (1853); and Comte Arthur deGobineau, *Essay on the Inequality of Human Races* (1853-1855). "deGobineau is commonly cited as the father of modern racism" (Roberts, 1995, p. 294).

From the idea that intermarriage of races somehow damages society and its institutions came the practices of lynching, separate drinking fountains, separate bus seating, and all the other ways by which the superiority of the white race was justified.[3] Christian philosophy contradicts such ideology. As stated by Roberts (1995):

> The official position of all major denominations in the United States is that Christianity and racism are mutually exclusive. Racism is viewed as a form of idolatry that is utterly incompatible with Christian theology. . . . Yet, despite the fact that racism and Christianity involve assumptions that are logically contradictory, the two ideologies have historically existed together and even been intertwined. (p. 295)

The Western world is one among other races that gave birth to racist ideology. The same Europeans that spread Christianity around the world also brought discrimination to America. It has affected and continues to affect the American experience, specifically members of minority communities as they seek full integration into American society. The quality of health care services minority populations receive is part of the process of integration that has been affected by racial discrimination.

RACIAL DISCRIMINATION
AND THE AMERICAN HEALTH CARE SYSTEM

Many studies have documented racial discrepancies in the quality of care Americans receive. Studies have found that if you are a white male you are more likely to receive better care than all other groups. In 1992 Charatz-Litt documented that legalized "segregation may have been outlawed in the 1960s, but the nation's vital statistics indicate that equality has yet to be achieved" (p. 717). Charatz-Litt did an overall assessment of health outcomes comparing blacks' and whites' state of health as reflected by the nation's vital statistics (1992). She concluded:

> As reflected in the current vital statistics for blacks in the United States, legal mandates have not been enough to combat the effects of racism. Institutions run primarily by white physicians continue to support racist activities. Only through education and persistence can Americans hope to change the current system and mold future generations. (p. 724)

What are some of the specific statistical realities faced by minorities in the United States? Becker and colleagues (1993) discovered that the black community "was at higher risk for cardiac arrest and subsequent death than the white community, even after we controlled for other variables" (1993, p. 606). Goldberg et al. (1992) found race and heart conditions to be statistically correlated. They discovered discrepancies in the number of coronary artery bypass graft surgery that males and females, blacks and whites received. For patients insured by Medicare (therefore all having similar access to health care services) the differences in receiving this procedure were great (whites

27.1 for 10,000; white males 40.4; white females 16.2; blacks 7.6; black males 9.3; black females 6.4) (p. 1473). These statistical differences were even more acute in the Southeast region of the nation.

Another example of differences in care received based on race categories was found by Sherman, Cody, and Solanchick (1993). "Black patients were 40 percent more likely than white patients to have a Kt/V less than 1.0 (45.6 percent of black patients v 32.5 percent of white patients, P = 0.038). Racial disparities in dialysis delivery exist, the causes and consequences of which need to be addressed" (pp. 632-633). Sehgal (2003) recently confirmed that even when concerted efforts are applied overall to improve the quality of care given to all patients, race and sex continue to be variables presenting disparities in health outcomes for hemodialysis patients. Sehgal (2003) confirmed that hemodialysis patients who happen to be black receive a type of care that produces more risks and poorer health outcomes. The same holds true for female patients at large. "Quality improvement efforts have a variable impact on race and sex disparities in health outcomes" (Sehgal, 2003, p. 1000). Minorities suffer from heart and kidney conditions at a greater rate than whites and from other medical disparities.

When researching the incidence of periodontitis, University of Michigan researchers discovered that race is a significant factor. Even when controlling for other variables, race continued to be a determinant for poorer oral health (Borrell et al., 2003).

The relation of patient race to care levels is clearly delineated by Carey and Mills Garrett:

> The relation of patient race to outcomes from and care for low back pain is complex. Blacks have slightly worse functional status than whites on presentation and at follow-up assessment. Blacks receive less intense diagnostic and treatment approaches from MDs, although the severity of their impairment is at least as great. (2003, p. 394)

Health care providers' preconceived notions influence every aspect of a patient's care. Hence, it is not surprising that race and sex negatively affect health outcomes.

Mental health for nonwhite populations is also an issue. According to the U.S. Department of Health and Human Services:

Minorities are less likely than whites to receive needed services and more likely to receive poor quality of care. By not receiving effective treatment, they have greater levels of disability in terms of lost workdays and limitations in daily activities. Further, minorities are overrepresented among the nation's most vulnerable populations, which have higher rates of mental disorders and more barriers to care. Taken together, these disparate lines of evidence support the finding that minorities suffer a disproportionately high disability burden from unmet mental health needs. (U. S. Department of Health and Human Services, 2001)

Iijima Hall (1997) writes: "With the changing demographics occurring in the United States, psychology must make substantive revisions in its curriculum, training, research, and practice" (p. 642). For Bernal and Castro (1994) the solution to the crisis in quality psychological care for nonwhite populations will be found in the "preparation for cultural competency rather than an introductory exposure to culture" of the providers (p. 797).

Racial Discrimination and the Four-Part Medical System

Physicians want to heal the patient's identified illness or condition. The whole system focuses on results. Health care practitioners are trained in a system driven by a four-part process: history taking, diagnosis (including all types of medical tests), treatment plan (including medications and therapeutic interventions), and evaluation (determining if the treatment plan was or was not effective). All four steps head in the same direction; to identify the culprit in the medical condition, and find a way to eliminate, ameliorate, or control this problem. The more elusive the problem, the greater the challenge. Medical researchers are at the peak of the medical pyramid when they devote their whole careers to pursuing answers for conditions that bewilder medical practitioners. But what can a nurse or physician do when the problem that is contributing to the health outcome cannot be seen, smelled, touched, or tested by any diagnostic tool? How can health care providers deal with a condition that is not easily perceived when taking the patient's medical history when it is not accounted for by the diagnostic models available, missed by the treatment plan, and can only be evaluated as part of a statistical process that ignores the individual patient?

Data showing discrepancies in incidence, care, and prognosis between blacks and whites suffering from hypertension are a longstanding mystery. Recently Brondolo and colleagues (2003) did a meta-analysis of published studies pertaining to hypertension with race as a significant variable altering health outcomes. Their conclusion was that "perceived racism" seemingly plays a crucial role, and they recommended further study of this variable in a more detailed fashion.

This is the case with racism; it is missed by all diagnostic tools but still has a pervasive influence on health outcomes. In a recently published study by Mandelblatt et al. (2003) regarding breast cancer patients, long-term outcomes in older cancer survivors were more about perceptions than patterns of care. "[T]he processes of care, and not the therapy itself, are the most important determinants of long-term quality of life in older women" (p. 863). They continue,

> women who perceived high levels of ageism or felt that they had no choice of treatment reported significantly more bodily pain, lower mental health scores, and less general satisfaction. These same factors, as well as high perceived racism, were significantly associated with diminished satisfaction with the medical care system. (p. 863)

The implications here are great, regardless of how well the treatment system works or the quality of the health care professionals and medical facilities. A key factor determining health outcomes is the patients' perception of how health care providers and systems view them in terms of race, age, and social status.

Patients' perceptions will be based on their interactions with health care providers and systems. These interactions are largely controlled by the health care system, rather than patients. What can a health care provider do to positively affect interactions with patients in order to promote health and healing?

CASE STUDIES

The elusive process of identifying racial prejudice is best taught via case studies. This method provides a multilayered discussion fed by a variety of opinions and experiences. This section presents three cases, under the sole control of the health care provider, which deal with issues of diversity. The focus is on the individual provider instead of administrators. This does not imply that there are no systemic approaches that could be used in each of these cases. All three could be analyzed from an administrative, institutional perspective.

The cases focus on helping the individual health care provider become aware of the subtle, mostly undetectable tentacles and pervasive influence of discrimination in the health care context. Class discussion will be facilitated by the four sections of each case presentation: (1) The Case Presentation; (2) Readings, Concepts, and Ideas for Discussing the Case; (3) Questions for Discussing This Case; and (4) Objectives.

The first case reflects whether people really have control over what they say, when they say it, and how they say it. The second case emphasizes the pervasiveness and nearly undetectable nature of prejudice. The last case focuses on the need to be aware of prejudice. How will each health care provider respond to the crisis presented by prejudice and racism in the context of a diverse population that *requires* intercultural communication?

You Control What You Say

Mental assessment of an infant-mother dyad; is the child properly attached?

A middle-class Puerto Rican mother with medical insurance provided by her employer brings her eighteen-month-old toddler in for a regular checkup.

HEALTH CARE PROVIDER: What brings you to our clinic today? How can I be of help?

MOTHER: My daughter Elizabeth, when fully awake and having been fed, seems to cry a lot.

HP: What do you mean? Do you suspect a particular condition? What have you observed?

M: Well, I want her to learn to be more in control of herself. She seems to want to be close to me all the time and cries whenever she needs something. I am concerned about her emotional development and overt attachment to me as her mom. Anyway, I cannot be there always. What can I do?

HP: Let me take a look at the child.

A complete physical is undertaken, a complete history recorded, vaccinations are given, and the doctor puzzles about how to address the mother's concerns.

HP: It seems to me that there is nothing wrong with your child. Crying is a normal way for toddlers to communicate with others.

M: But I need some way to control the child because I do not want her to develop into a disobedient child. I want her to learn to control herself and not always cry when she wants something. What can I do to promote this?

HP: I believe you need to change your expectations of how a child behaves. It is normal for a child to cry—she is a separate self that expresses herself independently from your own expectations.

If you were the HP what would you say to that mother? To prepare you for this task please read the following excerpts from authorities in the field of attachment behavior, which is part of mental health and self-identity development.

Readings, Concepts, and Ideas for Discussing the Case

Now evaluate the case and develop alternative approaches. First read what an expert on multicultural self-identity development has to say about individual identity. Richard Dana, Professor Emeritus, University of Arkansas, Fayetteville, is an authority in this area with over 100 published articles.

> Our knowledge of self-concept stems almost exclusively from research on Anglo Americans, individuals of the dominant culture in American society. The self for this population has firm boundaries that enclose what has been described as self-contained individualism, or egocentrism, characterized by personal control and a self-concept that excludes other persons (Sampson, 1985, 1988). Until recently it was assumed by most social scientists that the self-concept of persons from other cultures could be defined similarly. One obvious result of this assumption was that persons from other cultures have typically appeared as deficient in self-esteem as indicated by personality measures.

> In describing the identity of persons with non-European origins, it is necessary to consider an extended, or sociocentric self (Sampson, 1985, 1988). This augmented self is responsible and obligated to a variety of other persons who are affected by the individual's actions and have to be considered in all decision-making and problem-solving situations. (Dana, 1993, p. 11)

The second authority is an expert in attachment behavior of Puerto Ricans in comparison with European Americans. The reading comes from a book dealing with the complexities involved in a mother-child dyad's attachment behaviors and the influence of culture in determining outcomes and expectations (Harwood, Miller, and Lucca, 1995).

> As suggested earlier, the demands of proper demeanor vary with age, gender, and social status. For all children in Puerto Rico, it includes being *obediente* (obedient), *tranquilo* (calm), and *amable* (polite, gentle, kind). A child who is *intranquilo* (restless) lacks capacity to attend to other's needs and wishes, and a child who is disobedient or impolite defies authority. Such children are *malcriados,* a term that can be translated not only as "poorly brought up" but also as "ill-mannered." (p. 99)

> Like the Anglo mothers, Puerto Rican mothers expressed concern that their children [toddlers twelve to twenty-four months old] learn to control negative tendencies toward aggression, greed and egotism. However, whereas Anglo mothers tended to focus on these factors hindering self-maximization, Puerto Rican mothers appeared to view them as drives giving rise to behaviors that can threaten relationships and one's standing in the community. (p. 107)

The last authority cited is a European experimenter group from the Center for Child and Family Studies, Leiden University, the Netherlands.

> Contrary to our expectations, the more frequently mothers ignored their infants' crying bouts in the first nine-week period, the less frequently their infants cried in the following nine-week period, even if intervening variables like earlier crying and synchronous responsiveness were controlled for. "Benign neglect" of fussing may stimulate the emergent abilities in infants to cope with mild distress. (van Ijzendoorn and Hubbard, 2000, p. 391)

Questions for Discussing This Case

1. What are the reported aims of Puerto Rican mothers for their children? How do you compare these aims to that of the majority culture?
2. Do the aims of the mother in this case fit the aims Puerto Ricans are supposed to have? If yes, what does this mean? If no, how so?
3. Is it useful to learn about the general characteristics of people from various ethnic, racial, and cultural backgrounds? How can you use this knowledge?

Objectives

1. Develop awareness that there is more diversity in perspectives within any one group (i.e., Puerto Ricans) than between groups (i.e., European Americans and Puerto Ricans).
2. Develop awareness that as a HP your perception of your patients has an impact on your treatment.
3. Develop awareness that all cultural generalizations are made within the HP's own framework of cultural values and expectations. The practitioner's own expectation of the "normal" way for toddlers to act will guide his or her interventions.

You Cannot Control What You Were Taught

This case has several layers. Concentrate on the aspects that were under the control of the surgeon. All human interactions begin with categories of normalcy and truth, as well as each person's norms of propriety and behavior. Communication is not just "saying your piece." It involves trying to understand the definitions, rules of propriety, and understandings of "normalcy" each person has.

For the most part, most of these levels of communication occur at a subconscious level.

A twenty-five-month-old male child is brought to the emergency room at the hospital. The mother speaks mainly Spanish and understands very little English. The child's hand was severely damaged in a car accident. His right hand was trapped between the car seat and the door. Glass and metal almost totally severed three fingers. After examination it is determined that the fingers are beyond repair and have to be amputated. The surgeon comes to the hospital room to secure informed consent for the surgery. After trying to communicate with her limited knowledge of Spanish, she determines she will need the help of a translator. Following the hospital's protocol she checks the hospital's employee translator list and identifies a bilingual housekeeping employee who speaks Spanish. The surgeon explains the situation to the mother while the housekeeping employee translates. The mother signs the appropriate papers and the child is taken for surgery.

After surgery the mother sees that the child's right hand is missing three fingers and begins screaming uncontrollably. Upon investigation the housekeeping employee said: "It was too harsh to tell the mother that the three fingers were to be amputated. I had to give her some hope. I translated that the surgeon would try to save the fingers."

Readings, Concepts, and Ideas for Discussing the Case

The first reading comes from "Ethics, Rights, and Responsibilities," a document from the Joint Commission on Accreditation of Health-Care Organizations (2002).

Overview

The goal of the ethics, rights, and responsibilities is to improve care, treatment, services, and outcomes by recognizing and respecting the rights of each patient and by conducting business relationships with patients and the public in an ethical manner. Care, treatment, and services are provided in a way that respects and fosters dignity, autonomy, positive self-regard, civil rights, and involvement of patients. Care, treatment, and services consider the strengths, weaknesses, and resources of the patient; the relevant demands of his or her environment; and the requirements and expectations of the providers and those they serve.

"Proposed Revisions to Rights for Hospitals; Ethics, Rights, and Responsibilities;" Standard RI.2.2. "Patients have a Right to Effective Communication." Elements of Performance for RI.2.2.

The hospital respects the right and need of patients for effective communication. Written information provided is appropriate to the age, understanding, and language of the patient. The hospital provides for interpretation (including translation services) as necessary.

The second reading comes from specialists in bilingualism and intergenerational change. In 1985 McLaughlin and Stevenson reported what U.S. census information from 2000 confirms. For first generation immigrants, primary language is more than just a means to communicate; it represents an important part of their identity. This generation has difficulties with English and attributes great importance to their mother tongue; the second generation becomes proficient in English and deemphasizes their mother tongue.

> Many parents of minority-language children, for example, may feel exploited by the dominant society, yet may desire their children to learn the language so that the children have the opportunity to advance economically. At the same time, members of ethnolinguistic minority groups may desire that their children retain the first language. Languages have more than a mere pragmatic role in people's lives: They also have symbolic connotations. For older immigrants especially, the first language is likely to symbolize the home, friends, religion, warmth, and leisure; whereas, the second language is the language of the workplace and the language used to deal with impersonal authorities and institutions. If this is the case, it is easy to understand why the older generations cling to the first language and seeks to maintain it in their children's speech. (p. 187)

The third reading for this case comes from Gerald R. Winslow (1996). He discusses the variety of languages within the medical world. In a sense, health care has become multilingual.

> I have not argued that the metaphors of war, law, and business have no useful place in health care. Clearly, they do. What is equally clear, I think, is that the metaphors of ministry should not be lost. They can still provide powerful reminders of the central purpose of health care, to serve those who are in need. Finding fresh ways to keep the language of ministry alive should be a welcome task for those of us who find in health care an opportunity for spiritual service. (p. 29)

Questions for Discussing This Case

1. What values guided the surgeon in determining how communication takes place? What values did the mother have to cling to the Spanish language?
2. What values were guiding the housekeeping employee in determining how to translate for the desperate mother?
3. What could the surgeon have done to prevent this situation from taking place? What does the language of ministry demand of the health care provider?

Objectives

1. Develop awareness that humans are constantly ruled by subconscious norms of propriety and demeanor that are often not brought to the surface.
2. Develop awareness that all humans are bound by their subconscious, unspoken definitions of what is "normal." When interacting with others, these definitions of "normalcy" guide one's communication. When crossing from one cultural setting to another within the context of human communication, health care providers are responsible for becoming aware of the other person's concepts of "normal communication" and rules of propriety.
3. Develop awareness of the difficulties of communicating across cultures and the additional difficulty when a different language and translators are involved.

Treating Health Care Providers for Prejudice

This case comes from a *Los Angeles Times* article by Sonia Nazario.

> Althea Alexander broke her arm. At Los Angeles County-USC Medical Center the attending resident told her to hold her arm the way she usually holds a can of beer Saturday night. Alexander, who is black, exploded. "What are you talking about?" she demanded. "Do you think I'm a welfare mother?" The white resident shrugged: "Well, aren't you?" Wrong. Alexander was a

top official at the USC School of Medicine, where the resident was studying. (1993, p. A1)

Readings, Concepts, and Ideas for Discussing the Case

Rotheram and Phinney (1987) discuss how dominant culture often believes that its norms define the norm for everyone.

> The differences in behavioral norms, expectations, values, and behavior patterns that distinguish groups are less frequently recognized by Whites because most of their contacts are with other Whites, or their contacts with non-Whites are in contexts in which White norms prevail. Thus many majority group children [and adults] are not even aware that they belong to an ethnic group. (p. 17)

The second reading comes from a recent publication by Balsa and McGuire (2003). They discuss the fact that prejudice and stereotyping have a direct negative impact on health outcomes for patients from minority populations. The mental constructs that are often unconscious manifestations of being members of the majority group are presented as contributing factors for producing health disparities between minority patients and white patients.

> Disparities in health can result from the clinical encounter between a doctor and a patient. This paper studies three possible mechanisms: prejudice of doctors in the form of being less willlng to interact with members of minority groups, clinical uncertainty associated with doctors' differential interpretation of symptoms from minority patients or from doctors' distinct priors across races, and stereotypes doctors hold about health-related behavior of minority patients. Within a unified conceptual framework, we show how all three can lead to disparities in health and health services use. We also show that the effect of social policy depends critically on the underlying cause of disparities. (p. 89)

The third reading comes from the Association of American Medical Colleges, and the alarming conclusions of the study are discussed by Deborah Danoff (1999). The study, originally published by the

New England Journal of Medicine, reveals in crude detail that physicians, as representatives of the health care establishment, do contribute to the disparities in care received by minorities and women.

> Despite the medical profession's best efforts to promote diversity and cultural competence in its ranks, a new study published in the Feb. 25 [1999] *New England Journal of Medicine* reveals that racial and gender bias may still play an insidious role in influencing physicians' decision making. The study's authors report that women and blacks presenting with chest pain were almost two times as likely as white men not to be referred for cardiac catheterization.

> Using modern multimedia technology, a team of researchers from Georgetown University School of Medicine, the RAND Corporation, and the University of Pennsylvania, led by Georgetown associate professor of Medicine Kevin Schulman, MD, set out to address the question of bias in physicians' recommendations, while controlling for factors that had proved problematic for previous such studies, like age, risk factors, and even patient personality.

> The 720 physicians participating in the survey were randomly assigned to interact with a video of one of eight patient actors—two black men, two black women, two white men, and two white women. The "patients" read from one of three identical scripts, and physicians were given the same "medical history" and "personal information" regardless of the actor. "Race and sex differences in heart disease management had previously been reported in epidemiological studies, but it had remained unclear whether physicians had contributed to the disparities," commented Dr. Schulman. "Now we know that they do."

Questions for Discussing This Case

1. Which side of this story do you identify with the most?
2. Was the resident maliciously trying to put Althea down? If so, for what purpose? If not, how do you explain his words?
3. What can you do to prevent yourself from making assumptions like the resident did? Do you think the resident had a personal relationship with many people like Althea?

Objectives

1. Develop awareness of the need to have a personal strategy for growth.
2. Develop awareness of the need to reach beyond comfort zones and make friends with people who are different from you by visiting their places of comfort.
3. Develop awareness of the complexity and difficulty a dominant culture has when trying to understand what it means to be in the minority.

In general, minorities spend a lot of their time outside the boundaries of their cultural upbringing. They may have two or more cultures, and have learned to survive and perform outside their personal comfort zone. For them, intercultural relations are more about necessity than choice. Medical professionals need to look outside their own cultural boundaries and assumptions and develop intercultural communication skills by becoming acquainted with persons from a variety of languages and cultures.

A DIVERSE VISION OF WHOLENESS IN HEALTH CARE

This brief discussion about diversity, health, and wholeness has only scratched the surface of the issues involved in dealing with diversity within the context of the American health care system. However, it can help health care providers come to an appreciation of the complexity and challenges of diversity, especially as we seek to provide wholeness to patients. We need to step beyond our comfort zone and be willing to acknowledge differences in whatever context we may find ourselves. This challenge is not just a perspective but a responsibility if we take seriously our calling to address a person as a whole individual.

As a Christian living within a Western, early twenty-first century American framework influenced by Puerto Rican-Hispanic culture and an ordained minister teaching at a health sciences university in Southern California (who enjoys the prerogatives of being male) I have learned a great deal about diversity and spirituality from Hindu,

Buddhist, Confucian, and Muslim students and other students from various religious backgrounds and from a variety of disciplines.

Students have brought to life the meaning of integrating spirituality into health care to make health care not solely or mainly an industry but, as argued by Winslow (1996), a ministry; a ministry *to* a diverse population *by* a diverse population. Diversity that lives up to the WHO standards needs to further the state of being complete by making patients whole. The Bible says it best—"The thief comes only to steal and kill and destroy; I have come that they may have life, and have it to the full" (John 10:10, NIV).

NOTES

1. Chinese, Japanese, and Filipinos in general seem to have lower incidence rates than whites (Jenkins and Kagawa-Singer, 1994). However, Chinese Americans are at higher risk for cancer of the liver and esophagus (Barringer, Gardner, and Levin, 1993). Studies of the role of immigration in relation to health reveals significant findings. D. B. Thomas found an increased risk for breast, prostate, colon, rectal, and pancreatic cancer among Japanese and Chinese who immigrated to the United States (Thomas, 1979). These studies help us understand the importance of diversity as health care providers.

2. Americans have viewed diversity in both positive and negative ways. There is a tendency to value uniformity and integration rather than diversity. In 1963 Nathan Glazer and Daniel Moynihan offered their perspective on the "melting pot." They said that the notion of the unprecedented mixture of ethnic and religious groups in American life becoming homogeneous has outlived its usefulness and credibility. Meanwhile the persistent fact of ethnicity demands attention, understanding, and accommodation (Glazer and Moynihan, 1963).

3. Attitudes against interracial marriages further contribute to this process of discrimination. In 1993 there were 246,000 black-white married couples in this country while 50,000,000 marriages took place within the same year (U. S. Bureau of the Census, 1993). This number seems to suggest social forces that go against the idea of interracial marriage. From a legal point of view, it was not until a U. S. Supreme Court decision (*Loving* v. *Commonwealth of Virginia*) in 1967, that interracial marriage was legalized (Rosenblatt, Karis, and Powell, 1995).

REFERENCES

Balsa, A.I. and McGuire, T.G. (2003). Prejudice, clinical uncertainty and stereotyping as sources of health disparities. *Journal of Health Economy,* 22(1):89-116.
Barringer, H.R., Gardner, J.J., and Levin, M.J. (1993). *Asians and Pacific Islanders in the United States.* New York: Russell Sage Foundation.

Becker, L.B., Han, B.H., Meyer, P.M., Wright, F.A., Rhodes, K.V., Smith, D.W., and Barrett, J. (1993). Racial differences in the incidence of cardiac arrest and subsequent survival. The CPR Chicago Project. *New England Journal of Medicine,* 329(9):600-606.

Bernal, M.E. and Castro, F.G. (1994). Are clinical psychologists prepared for service and research with ethnic minorities? Report of a decade of progress. *American Psychologist,* 49(9):797-805.

Borrell, L.N., Taylor, G.W., Borgnakke, W.S., Nyquist, L.V., Woolfolk, M.W., Allen, D.J., and Lang, W.P. (2003). Factors influencing the effect of race on established periodontitis prevalence. *Journal of Public Health Dentistry,* 63(1):20-29.

Brondolo, E., Rieppi, R., Kelly, K.P., and Gerin, W. (2003). Perceived racism and blood pressure: A review of the literature and conceptual and methodological critique. *Annals of Behavioral Medicine,* 25(1):55-65.

Carey, T.S. and Mills Garrett, J. (2003). The relation of race to outcomes and the use of health care services for acute low back pain. *Spine,* 28(4):390-394.

Charatz-Litt, C. (1992). A chronicle of racism: The effects of the white medical community on black health. *Journal of the National Medical Association,* 84(8):717-725.

Dana, R.H. (1993). *Multicultural assessment perspectives for professional psychology.* Boston: Allyn & Bacon.

Glazer, N. and Moynihan, D.P. (1963). *Beyond the melting pot: The Negroes, Puerto Ricans, Jews, Italians, and Irish of New York City.* Cambridge, MA: MIT Press.

Goldberg, K.C., Hartz, A.J., Jacobsen, S.J., Krakauer, H., and Rimm, A.A. (1992). Racial and community factors influencing coronary artery bypass graft surgery rates for all 1986 Medicare patients. *Journal of the American Medical Association,* 267(11):1473-1477.

Harwood, R.L., Miller, J.G., and Lucca Irizarry, N. (1995). *Culture and attachment: Perceptions of the child in context.* New York: The Guilford Press.

Iijima Hall, C.C. (1997). Cultural malpractice; The growing obsolescence of psychology with changing U.S. populations. *American Psychologist,* 52(6):642-651.

Jenkins, C.N.H. and Kagawa-Singer, M. (1994). Cancer. In N.W.S. Zane, D.T. Takeuchi, and K.N.J. Young (Eds.), *Confronting critical health issues of Asian and Pacific Islander Americans* (pp. 105-147). Thousand Oaks, CA: Sage Publications.

Joint Commission on Accreditation of Health-Care Organizations (2002). Ethics, Rights, and Responsibilities: Preamble, and Proposed Revisions to Rights for Hospitals; Ethics, Rights, and Responsibilities; Standard RI.2.2, Patients have a right to effective communication, and Elements of Performance for RI.2.2, retrieved from <www.jcaho.org> on March 2, 2003.

Jordan, W.D. (1968). *White over black.* Baltimore: Penguin.

Kelsey, G.D. (1965). *Racism and the Christian understanding of man.* New York: Scribner.

Kennedy, J.F. (1964). *A nation of immigrants.* Revised and enlarged with introduction by Robert F. Kennedy. New York: Harper and Row.

Mandelblatt, J.S., Edge, S.B., Meropol, N.J., Senie, R., Tsangaris, T., Grey, L., Peterson, B.M. Jr., Hwang, Y.T., Kerner, J., and Weeks, J. (2003). Predictors of long-term outcomes in older breast cancer survivors: Perceptions versus patterns of care. *Journal of Clinical Oncology,* 21(5):855-863.

McLaughlin, B. and Stevenson, A. (1985). *Second-language acquisition in childhood:* Volume 2, *School-age children,* Second edition. Hillsdale, NJ: Lawrence Erlbaum Associates.

Mosse, G.L. (1978). *Toward a final solution: A history of European racism.* New York: Harper and Row.

Nazario, S. (1993). Treating doctors for prejudice. *Los Angeles Times,* December 20, Section A:1, pp. 36-37.

Niebuhr, R. (1941, 1964). *The nature and destiny of man: A Christian interpretation.* New York: Charles Scribner's Sons.

Race and gender bias in medicine: What educators can do (1999). *Reporter,* Association of American Medical Colleges, Vol. 8; (8), May.

Roberts, K.A. (1995). *Religion in sociological perspective,* Third edition. Belmont, CA: Wadsworth Publishing Company.

Rosenblatt, P.C., Karis, T.A., and Powell, R.D. (1995). *Multiracial couples: Black and white voices.* Thousand Oaks: Sage Publications.

Rotheram, M.J. and Phinney, J.S. (1987). Introduction: Definitions and perspectives in the study of children's ethnic socializations. In J.S. Phinney and M.J. Rotheram (Eds.), *Children's ethnic socialization: Pluralism and development* (pp. 10-31). Newbury Park, CA: Sage.

Sehgal, A.R. (2003). Impact of quality improvement efforts on race and sex disparities in hemodialysis. *Journal of the American Medical Association,* 289(8):996-1000.

Sherman, R.A., Cody, R.P., and Solanchick, J.C. (1993). Racial differences in the delivery of hemodialysis. *American Journal of Kidney Disease,* (6):632-634.

Staum, M.S. (2000). Paris ethnology and the perfectibility of "races." *Canadian Journal of History,* 35(3):453-473.

The Gallup Organization (2003). Poll topics and trends, immigration, retrieved February 28, 2003 from <www.gallup.com>.

Thomas, D.B. (1979). Epidemiologic studies of cancer in minority groups in the Western United States. *National Cancer Institute Monographs,* 3, 103-113.

U. S. Bureau of the Census (1993). *Statistical abstract of the United States.* Washington, DC: Government Printing Office.

U. S. Census Bureau (2001). Population by race and Hispanic or Latino origin, for all ages, for the United States: 2000. Department of Commerce: Internet Release date April 2, 2001, <www.census.gov>.

U. S. Department of Health and Human Services (2001). Mental health: Culture, race, and ethnicity: A supplement to mental health: A report of the Surgeon General. *Executive Summary*. Author.

van Ijzendoorn, M.H. and Hubbard, F.O. (2000). Are infant crying and maternal responsiveness during the first year related to infant-mother attachment at fifteen months? *Attachment of Human Development,* 2(3):371-391.

Winslow, G.R. (1996). Minding our language: Metaphors and biomedical ethics. In E.E. Shelp (Ed.), *Secular bioethics in theological perspective* (pp. 19-30). Boston: Kluwer Academic Publishers.

World Health Organization (1948). WHO definition of health. Found at the Preamble to the Constitution of the World Health Organization as adopted by the International Health Conference, New York, June 19-22, 1946; signed on July 22, 1946, by the representatives of 61 States (Official Records of the World Health Organization, no. 2, p. 100) and entered into force on April 7, 1948.

Chapter 8

Working with Difficult Patients: Spiritual Care Approaches

Leigh Aveling
Siroj Sorajjakool
Reginald Pulliam

OBJECTIVES

1. To describe experiences of patients and health care professionals in dealing with difficult situations.
2. To attempt to conceptualize "difficult" patients in clinical settings by exploring characteristics, interpretation, and the dynamics of relationships.
3. To explore methods of intervention in dealing with difficult patients.
4. To provide an understanding of spiritual care within the context of difficult patients/situations.

INTRODUCTION

An eighteen-year-old high school senior living in a boarding school dormitory complained of a headache, and later collapsed in the shower. Upon her arrival at the nearest community hospital it was discovered that the lack of medical resources precluded treatment. Therefore, the patient was transferred to the regional trauma center where she was diagnosed with meningitis. After the first forty-eight hours passed with no sign of improvement, a conference was held with the family and treatment team. Supporting the family in every way they could, the team wanted to prepare the family for a worst-case scenario.

Medically, there was minimal confirmation that the patient was alive. There was no evidence of brain activity and negligible brain-stem function. The family demanded that everything be done to preserve life. Although extremely sympathetic, the team wanted the family to be realistic. After consultation with the hospital ethics team, the family was told that the patient met the criteria for brain death. Because the patient was a minor, and a foreign-exchange student and her family lived outside the United States, she lacked the type of insurance needed for this type of catastrophic coverage involving extensive long-term care. Therefore, the family needed to cover the expense. Bed, ventilator, and ancillary treatments needed to maintain the patient were extremely expensive. The bill after a week was over $100,000. The family was approached about turning off life support, but they wanted and needed more time. Some of the staff began to view the family as somewhat noncompliant and difficult to deal with. Others were sympathetic, but felt that the family was becoming difficult to work with.

After another week of meeting the criteria for brain death, the family agreed to turn off life support, but only after they were able to bring in pastors from their church to pray over the patient. The team agreed.

The next day the hospital chaplain walked by the patient's room. The curtains were drawn. He asked a somewhat skeptical social worker what was happening there. She replied that they were engaging in some weird chant. The chaplain listened carefully and recognized that the family was engaged in prayer in their native language. As the prayer ended, the nurse felt the patient squeeze her hand; another family member thought she saw the patient frown. Vital signs started to improve and within a few days the patient was able to converse. She was discharged to a rehabilitation facility, graduated at the end of the school year, maintained her grade point average despite her lengthy hospital stay, and graduated summa cum laude.

Because such miracles are rare, this scenario raises a very important question regarding patient care: How do we distinguish patients (and at times, their families) who are difficult from those who are not?

CONTEXTS

Most health care professionals have to deal with difficult patients at one time or another. In clinical settings such as a hospital, dealing with difficult patients is unavoidable since there is continuous interaction between the health care professional and patients, families and friends, and other staff members with various backgrounds and personalities. The goal of this chapter is to conceptualize difficult patients in clinical settings. The discussion of the difficult patient will be organized as follows:

1. description of characteristics,
2. description of an interpretive model of care,

3. description of relationship dynamics and implications,
4. intervention, and
5. the importance of spirituality to patient care.

Several scenarios will be interspersed within these sections and re-framed in a spiritual context along with suggestions for application.

Characteristics

George, a young man in his early twenties, has sickle-cell anemia and needs pain control medications. He is in pain and angry. He wants Demerol and asks his nurse fourteen times in thirty minutes to give him a shot. She refuses because administering more medication would suppress his breathing and could be life threatening. George has a criminal record and is well-known by police and medical professionals in his community. On numerous occasions he has been arrested for drug possession, particularly Demerol. Because of his addiction, George manipulates his supply with frequent visits to hospital emergency rooms. He throws tantrums when doctors refuse to renew his prescriptions or provide him with his drug fixes. Since George's hostile outbursts prevent him from receiving appropriate treatment as perceived by his caregivers, overworked and suspicious physicians do not want to deal with him and want him out of their way.

What is a difficult patient? The empirical literature suggests that particular attributes are indicative of "good" versus "bad" patients and can be identified by health care staff within the first twenty-four hours of hospitalization (Ritvo, 1963). "Good" characteristics include, but are not limited to, emotional stability, cheerfulness, controlled feelings and anxiety levels, communicability, appreciativeness, conformity, and consideration. Negative attributes include emotional instability, hostility, aggressiveness, impatience, overly dependent or independent behavior, manipulativeness, stubbornness, and noncompliance (Sarosi, 1968; Smith and Steindler, 1983). Despite such representations, these attributes are not independent. They exist as part of a larger system of beliefs that seem to clash when patients and health care providers have opposing perspectives regarding the nature of health care (MacGregor, 1967; Smith and Steindler, 1983). Roadblocks to desired treatment goals come in various forms: an angry patient refuses to take medication; family members refuse to accept the dying process of a loved one; a religious person refuses treatment on the basis of her faith. Hence the term difficult is relative to alignment between the goals of patients and caregivers.

Interpretation

How treatment goals and patient behavior are perceived involves a significant interpretive process. Clinicians' interpretations of patient responses play an important role. Because time is a scarce commodity for many in the medical field, a patient who absorbs a great deal of time on what the clinician considers nonemergent matters will possibly be viewed as difficult.

Are patients merely trying to survive, or are the observed behaviors a baseline of everyday behavior? Perhaps they are indeed facing a crisis, or feel that they are. This perceived crisis has a significant impact on subsequent emotional expression. Emotional reactions vary depending on how patients view their crisis. If patients feel stressed and afraid, they shift to survival mode. Physiological changes, such as an increase in heartbeat and narrowing of pupils, may be apparent. When patients are in survival mode, emotional reactivity, which is a type of defense mechanism, is activated. Emotional reactivity is often expressed in the form of denial, or even regression. In such cases, reactive patients may regress to a type of behavior that seems childlike, oppositional, or dependent. Patients use defense mechanisms to help them cope with difficult situations.

Clinicians, particularly those working with such patients, may see these types of behaviors on a daily basis. What is an extreme situation for the patient may be a daily event for staff members. For instance, in response to a patient requesting to see his or her doctor, a nurse may respond, "the doctor will be with you shortly," knowing that it could be hours. The conflict in interpretation is most noticeable under these circumstances. How patients interpret their need may differ significantly from that of caregivers. The level of anxiety coupled with uncertainty regarding details and implications of the illness can lead patients to interpret the illness as a crisis. Howard Stone, professor of pastoral care and counseling, states accurately, "for a crisis to develop, a serious threat to self or family has to be perceived." He further explains:

> During a crisis, people's mental circuits become overloaded. They see the threat as incompatible with their precrisis pattern of thinking about themselves or their world. This overload of incompatible information sometimes called "cognitive dissonance," interferes with usual ways of planning and carrying out effective

actions. The cognitive dissonance, which results from people's appraisal of the threat inherent in an event, leads them first to try old and then new and different ways of eradicating the confusing feelings. (Stone, 1993, p. 25)

Although both patients and caregivers may wish to see the same ultimate result, interpretation may differ regarding the seriousness of the illness; further complicating the process and hindering caregivers from reaching the defined goal. Thus we may be compelled, as David Tracy has stated, "to find new ways of interpreting ourselves" (1987, p. 8).

John Brown

A reflection on a specific case from this model can help to deepen our existential understanding of this conceptualization of the difficult patient.

John Brown was recently diagnosed with leukemia and told that his prognosis was not good. In mentioning his grim outlook, however, the doctors did not want to take all hope away from him. They felt that if he knew he only had weeks to live, he would be too overwhelmed, but the social worker observed that John seemed to be aware of his situation.

At the request of his nurse a chaplain went to visit him. They talked about superficial things for a few moments. John appeared overwhelmed and tired. A chaplain asked if there was anything he could do and his response was a request for prayer. He said he had lots to think about and wanted some time to think. The chaplain prayed with him and left.

During psychosocial rounds some weeks later, the nurse shook her head in frustration. When John was awake he did not want to get out of bed. He would either give monosyllabic answers to questions or remain silent. His family provided little help. John's wife stated that he had been difficult to talk with for the thirty years of their marriage. For her, John's behavior was still the same, so why expect him to change?

As the weeks progressed, the social worker reported that John had stated that he wished to die. Apart from taking his medication, he did not want to bathe or eat. The team felt that he was noncompliant. He appeared to be depressed, with no will to participate in his treatment.

John refused to get out of bed until a persistent physical therapist coaxed him into a wheelchair and took him down the hall. That did not last very long. John wanted to remain in bed. Soon, even the persistent physical therapist could no longer persuade him to get out of bed. What was taking place here?

It slowly became apparent that there were tremendous family stresses in John's life. He seemed to be ambivalent about life. To add to his stress, his family was divided over his care. One family member wanted him listed as a DNR (do not resuscitate), while the others did not. Inevitably, John often experienced conflict. In the presence of his family he stated that he did not want to die. In contrast, when alone with various staff members he would report that he wanted to die, and was tired of the pain and suffering he was experiencing. John's ambivalence combined with his polarized family presented a challenge for the staff. Even consultation with the ethics team failed to bring closure to this dilemma.

A hospice chaplain recently made the remark that in his experience, the majority of patients die the same way they lived. In his ten years of hospice work he had never seen a deathbed conversion. Although this observation may be disputed by a few highly publicized conversions, he may be correct in making this assertion, especially when it comes to dealing with patients such as John. The hospice chaplain added that deathbed conversions rarely take place while a person is actively dying because they tend to be so heavily medicated, which precludes thinking in a rational manner.

A few months after his diagnosis, John was transferred to the intensive care unit. His family wanted the staff to keep him alive. John eventually settled the issue for everyone by dying peacefully in his sleep.

Difficult, or in John's case, noncompliant patients, especially during end-of-life episodes, are unlikely to change their baseline level of behavior. Clinicians tend to quickly identify patients with these behaviors as difficult after experiencing them a number of times.

An analysis of John Brown's case from the "goal-fulfillment" modality helps us better understand the difficulty experienced by John and his caregivers. John's caregivers perceived their goal as providing necessary medical care for him. His noncompliant behavior, in a subtle way, moved in the opposite direction of the goal they wished to achieve, to accept his condition and cope positively. But John did not cope positively. He "regressed." His depression seemed to symbolize the lack of progress in medical treatment. He became a difficult patient. The question of the validity of such an assumption from the medical professionals may be raised. Does depression mean failure? Is negative coping necessarily a bad thing? What about John? What was his goal? What did he really want? What does a dying person want? In suspending our moral judgment on John's desire, we realize that the medical professionals were working against everything that his depression had been telling him. Resistance emerged. There was a conflict in the desired outcome from both John and the world of medicine. But the medical professionals were not being perceived as difficult. John was. Whose goal has greater validity? The deeper issue underlying this conflict is spirituality. Perhaps spirituality is both the problem and the solution. Before discussing spirituality, relational dynamics and then practical solutions will be discussed.

Relational Dynamics/Implications

"I feel that I'm taking care of everyone, and I don't want to come back," stated a nurse while dealing with a difficult family situation. Some patients place excessive demands on caregivers' time, constantly ask for pain medication, and often use foul language. Another nurse mentioned that she feels stress whenever a call light goes on in a difficult patient's room. "Two or three unnecessary calls create an environment where I start to resent my patient." Still others comment that their own stress combined with abuse of the call light sometimes results in other patients receiving minimal basic care because they were forced to spend excessive time carefully documenting their every move. These examples illustrate that working in an environment with the physically ill may be emotionally stressful, resulting in the perception that a patient is difficult.

The "problem" patient is not merely the product of personality traits, but also results from an impaired patient-health care provider relationship (Juliana et al., 1997; MacGregor, 1967; Travelbee, 1971). Discrepancies in this relationship with regard to expectations in the therapeutic culture may lead to lack of communication and noncare of patients that is unethical and immoral (Maupin, 1995). Since reactions to illness seem to be culturally, socially, and individually determined (Hover and Juelsgaard, 1978) patients are often unprepared for the loss of autonomy and personal identity incurred upon entering the therapeutic or medical environment. Consequently, perceived coercion to conform to a different set of standards may lead to alienation and heightened defensive responses to novel, and at times, frightening circumstances. Part of the problem is faulty communication between patient and health care provider (Maxson, 1974). Incongruent self-other expectations may encourage further breakdowns in communication leaving patients feeling confused, angry, and unwilling to cooperate with professional staff. Over time, the cumulative and dynamic nature of this type of patient-health care provider interaction may cause responses that are detrimental to both patients and health care professionals (Robinson, 1976). To counter negative responses, several methods are suggested for the health care professional to implement during interactions with difficult patients.

Interventions

Management of patients labeled "difficult" can often be a daunting task for the health professional due to competing responsibilities. Mismanagement is often the result of poor patient-staff interaction. An important first step in the process of intervention is for the health care professional to maintain the proper perspective, which is to evaluate the context or situational determinants of patient behavior and not the patient as a person. This step is important because the perspective of the patient is often lost when we attempt to resolve problems based on patient responses (e.g., anger, noncompliance, etc.).

Other ways clinicians can deal effectively with such patients, particularly when there are varying opinions among family members, include: (1) scheduling family conferences with the multidisciplinary team, (2) maintaining hope as options are discussed and then examining the family dynamics for unfinished business, and (3) discussing the grief experience when a child or sibling has unfinished emotional business with a parent by scheduling time with the chaplain and/or physician for medical clarity. Difficult clinical situations with patients and families often represent a microcosm of daily life. Since patient/family responses vary, their interactions with staff raise concerns about the relationship among social, emotional, spiritual, cultural, and physical factors.

SPIRITUALITY AND DIFFICULT PATIENTS

From a spiritual perspective, there are no difficult patients. However, patients reframed in a spiritual context experience difficulty in finding existential meaning. Often, an underlying spiritual struggle exists behind the overt behavior of difficult patients. Difficult patients are often those who are unable to find meaning in their lives. Following the "goal-fulfillment" modality we can say that patients become difficult because the spiritual goal of discovering meaning has been hindered or suppressed by various factors in their lives. Meaning serves as a boundary function by giving organization to, seemingly, perplexing circumstances. The search for meaning "is our finitude," writes Paul Tillich, "in interdependence with the finitude of our world which drives us to search for ultimate reality" (1955, p. 14).

John stares into the face of death. It is a horrifying image with devastating implications. Martin Heidegger, an existentialist philosopher, understood this human dilemma. In the face of death, we are compelled to question and evaluate life, to look for its meaning. "The meaning of Being is—Time" (Rudiger Safranski, 1999, p. 148). But John has no time left and the struggle becomes more intense. It is not a fight for life. He is fighting for meaning. He is searching to make peace with death, the painful tranquility. But his quest, fueled by his unconscious awareness of the need for meaning, projected itself through depression and is interpreted as noncompliance.

Christine, an eighteen-year-old sickle-cell patient comes to the emergency room. She is in acute sickle-cell crisis. Part of this crisis is pain. She states that she is experiencing extreme pain and asks for Demerol.

The emergency room physician knows from previous experience with Christine that if he does not prescribe her drug of choice she will throw a tantrum. She will scream, curse, and make a scene, and the physician is tired. He has worked a long shift. There are other patients waiting to be seen. What should he do? He also knows that if he gives her a shot of Demerol it will relieve the pain almost instantly, but the relief will not be long lasting. The pain will return with a vengeance and Christine will be on her way to another emergency room asking for another shot. He decides that Christine meets the requirements for admission.

The staff on the cancer unit is also familiar with Christine and they are tired of her. During her numerous previous hospitalizations, they have found her to be manipulative and unpleasant. She constantly complains of pain. When asked about her pain level on a scale of 1 to 10 she replies 12, but then when no one is looking, she picks up the phone and orders a pizza. She complains incessantly. Finally, orders are written for a stronger medication. The complaints continue. She orders the nurse to remake her bed for the fifth time that morning and curses the nurse because her response was not immediate. Family members and visitors come and go at all hours. One of her friends is suspected of bringing in street drugs for her. She throws the telephone on the floor and breaks it. She refuses to get out of bed to use the rest room and soils herself rather than using a bedpan. The staff is weary and tired of her.

Christine is not only in pain but she has become a source of pain to others around her. Nurses have their goals and Christine is only one of the many patients they need to care for. Her demands hinder them from achieving their goals. Christine's personal goal is Demerol. Or is it? Could there be other goals such as the need to make sense of conflicting feelings, fear and anxiety, anger and resentment, faith and hope? Perhaps the complexity of the issue is beyond the grasp of an eighteen-year-old girl. How do we move beyond the behavior and address her soul? How can we provide spiritual care for Christine? Before addressing spiritual care for "difficult patients," some practical suggestions in dealing with this type of case are discussed.

Spiritual Care

How difficult a patient has become depends largely on the availability of time and the conscious decision of caregivers to deal with difficult situations. The question is, how much emotional and intellectual space has one created to contain "difficulty" in dealing with patients' anger, sadness, demands, or refusal? How much room does one have for restless souls grasping for light? To be realistic, the demands of work and the availability of time in the current health care system limit the space caregivers can offer to difficult patients. Moreover, the reality is that there are patients who are not agreeable. To deny this reality is to project artificiality that will only serve to depreciate authenticity of the level of care. Gerald May has succinctly articulated a prescription for sanity: "Do the best you can. Then wait" (1977, p. 114). Because that is all one can do, no more and no less.

Spiritual care requires commitment to the difficult task of creating mental and emotional space for restless souls, and a willingness to accept the fact that one's investment may yield no immediate results.

The journey toward meaning requires identification and acknowledgment of cognitive and emotional contributions to the existential questions of life. Meaning making is not an abstract intellectual endeavor. It is existential in nature. One cannot begin to make sense of one's experience unless one is able to name and become aware of feelings and thoughts that happen to the self. We cannot put the puzzle together unless we have all the pieces. Finding, naming, and owning these pieces need to take place. How can we facilitate this for difficult patients? D. W. Winnicott offers a helpful model. People who struggle for meaning when faced with life challenges may go through regressive behavior. But this regression may just be "a regression in search of true self" (cited by Ulanov, 2001, p. 49). In this quest, the presence of someone who will symbolically provide a holding in this critical moment, and provide a nonreactive presence in the midst of chaos, demands, anger, sadness, and unreasonableness is needed.

Reflecting on Winnicott's proposal, Ann Ulanov sees religion as a place where this holding can take place.

> Religion, I propose, can provide an environment that will support our going back for what we missed and so desperately need—feeling alive and real. . . . Religion points to the safe environment provided by the God who holds us in being. Through worship, the sacraments, and the counseling of a spiritual director, we may experience the safe holding that allows us to look into the gaps of dissociation between our bodies and psyches, into the terrors of ground falling away beneath us, into the moments of unreality when we feel the flicker of our uniqueness as persons faltering. Looking into such gaps, we may begin slowly, carefully to knit together what was broken apart. (2001, p. 49)

Several factors serve to create a holding space for difficult patients, enabling them to explore and organize ambiguous experiences. The conceptual aim is to free up a person so they can pay attention to the unconscious forces, feelings, thoughts, and reactions they are experiencing. This can be achieved in a number of ways.

A Nonreactive Presence

In a medical context, a screaming patient does so with the expectation that this behavior will result in attention to a need. Unfortunately, more often than not, a negative response is the result. Negative responses only further affirm a sense of self as chaotic and unworthy. The cumulative effects of situations like this produce in patients a preunderstanding of causal relation that says, "If I behave this way, I will receive that type of response." This causal relation imprinted on the unconscious self becomes the reality that a person lives with. A nonreactive presence alters this reality, changing the causal structure. A screaming person expects to be perceived as unworthy by the caregiver who responds negatively, and to be avoided. A nonreactive presence provides care as usual. With time, the difficult patient may construct a different reality. The patient's preconceived understanding of reality leaves no room for the acknowledgment of anger, an understanding that prejudges this feeling as negative and hence makes it impossible to integrate this emotion into the self. When a part of us that presents itself with strong emotion is judged as negative, it becomes impossible to put the pieces together, to make sense of these experiences. Awareness does not mean permitting screaming patients to do as they please. On the contrary, Jung (1984) has informed us that only through such an awareness can one learn to manage negative emotions.

A Listening Presence

Screaming, metaphorically speaking, is a desperate call for someone, a crying out to listen and to pay attention. In discussing spiritual care, Seward Hiltner (1955) suggests that the primary duty is to listen well. Caring is not about giving advice, providing guidance, or suggesting alternatives. It is about listening. Pastoral counselors who are trained to provide spiritual care for their clients understand this. Healing emerges by inviting clients to articulate what has been buried within their hearts. The process of conversation, particularly deep conversation, enables a person to have a better understanding of the self. It is a cyclical process in which deeper meaning of the self unfolds. According to David Tracy, "Conversation in its primary form is an exploration of possibilities in the search for truth" (1987, p. 20).

A Questioning Presence

A pastoral counselor once asked his supervisor how to deal with boredom while in session with clients. The supervisor's reply was most enlightening: "You are not curious enough. With enough curiosity, there is no boredom." Asking probing questions can elicit the unfolding of aspects of self that have remained buried or suppressed. First, one needs to be curious enough in an attempt to make sense of stories or ideas that difficult patients may be trying to communicate. Second, it is important to ask specific questions: "How are you doing?" will not get you to the deeper level. There is a qualitative difference between asking, "How do you feel today?" and "Were you hurt by his comments?" Third, be as concrete as possible during inquiry. Do not let the question remain abstract. Ask, "When did it happen? How did it happen?" The more concrete the conversation, the better a person becomes in making sense of his or her stories.

CONCLUSION

A difficult patient engenders a variety of characteristics perceived as prohibitive to effective treatment as defined by the health care professional. Treatment goals are relative to perception and interpretation of both the patients and the caregivers. In principle, goal alignment is the product of a collaborative effort between patients, their families, and clinical staff. This principle is also applied to spiritual care. A key provision of spiritual care is identification of the spiritual goal of patients. In their broadest sense, spiritual goals represent a quest for existential meaning incorporated in a process of discovery that varies by patient. A patient seems difficult because he or she has trouble organizing the life implications of a traumatic event such as physical illness as applied to self and others. Because the discovery of meaning is a personal journey, it is imperative for clinical staff to be compassionate and demonstrate a favorable attitude toward patients dealing with how to integrate the varying aspects of who they are (e.g., spiritual, physical, emotional, psychological, social) within the context of physical illness. Spiritual care requires understanding and a stable presence that listens.

GUIDED QUESTIONS

1. What is the relationship between attributes of difficult patients and belief systems?
2. What role does interpretation play when dealing with difficult situations?
3. In the case of John, what was his goal and what was the goal of the treatment team?
4. What are the four practical approaches one can employ in dealing with difficult situations?
5. What should one pay attention to when attempting to provide spiritual care for difficult patients?
6. Name three approaches you can use in providing spiritual care for difficult patients.

REFERENCES

Hiltner, S. (1955). *Preface to pastoral theology.* New York: Abingdon.

Hover, J. and Juelsgaard, N. (1978). The sick role reconceptualized. *Nursing Forum,* 17, 407-415.

Juliana, C. A., Orehowsky, S., Smith-Regojo, P., Sikora, S. M., Smith, P. A., Stein, D. K., Wagner, D. O., and Wolf, Z. R. (1997). Interventions used by staff nurses to manage "difficult" patients. *Holistic Nursing Practice,* 11(4), 1-26.

Jung, C. (1984). *Psychology and western religion.* Princeton, NJ: Princeton University Press.

MacGregor, F. C. (1967). Uncooperative patients: Some cultural interpretations. *American Journal of Nursing,* 67, 88-91.

Maupin, C. R. (1995). The potential for noncaring when dealing with difficult patients: Strategies for moral decision making. *Journal of Cardiovascular Nursing,* 9, 11-22.

Maxson, K. (1974). Assuming the patient role. *Perspectives in Psychiatric Care,* 12, 119-122.

May, G. (1977). *Simply sane: The spirituality of mental health.* New York: Crossroad.

Ritvo, M. M. (1963). Who are "good" and "bad" patients? *Modern Hospital,* 100, 79-81.

Robinson, L. (1976). *Psychological aspects of the care of hospitalized patients.* Philadelphia: F. A. Davis.

Safranski, R. (1999). *Martin Heidegger: Between good and evil.* Massachusetts: Harvard University Press.

Sarosi, G. M. (1968). A critical theory: The nurse as a fully human person. *Nursing Forum,* 7, 349-363.

Smith, R. J. and Steindler, E. M. (1983). The impact of difficult patients upon treaters: Consequences and remedies. *Bulletin of the Menninger Clinic,* 47, 107-116.

Stone, H. (1993). *Crisis counseling.* Minneapolis: Fortress.

Tagore, R. (1941). *Gitanjali.* New York: Scribner Poetry.

Tillich, P. (1955). *Biblical religion and the search for ultimate reality.* Chicago: University of Chicago Press.

Tracy, D. (1987). *Plurality and ambiguity: Hermeneutics, religion, hope.* Chicago: University of Chicago Press.

Travelbee, J. (1971). *Interpersonal aspects of nursing.* Philadelphia: F. A. Davis.

Ulanov, A. (2001). *Finding space: Winnicott, God, and psychic reality.* Louisville: Westminster John Knox Press.

Index